What's So Funny?
The Autobiography of a Professional
Schizophrenian, Artist, Singer, and Public Speaker

By Jude Mersereau

Library and Archives Canada Cataloguing in Publication

Title: What's so funny? : the autobiography of a professional schizophrenian, artist, public
   speaker and singer / by Jude Mersereau.
Other titles: Autobiography of a professional schizophrenian, artist, public speaker and singer
Names: Mersereau, Jude, 1966- author.
Identifiers: Canadiana 20210125330 | ISBN 9781927637371 (softcover)
Subjects: LCSH: Mersereau, Jude, 1966- | LCSH: Schizophrenics—Canada—Biography. | LCSH: Artists—
   Canada—Biography. | LCSH: Singers—Canada—Biography. | LCSH: Orators—Canada—Biography. | LCGFT:
   Autobiographies.
Classification: LCC RC514 .M47 2021 | DDC 616.89/80092—dc23

Bridgeross Communications
Dundas, Ontario, Canada
ISBN 978-1-927637-37-1

Table of Contents

To Georgie, the better half of Jeordy

Familial Interjection/Preface

Welcome to Jude's world. Yes, Jude's. We've known her as Judy, but she prefers her nom de plume here, as on her paintings and on stage as well.

So what's in a name? Lots, especially in the world of mental patients where medical labels play such a part in where you live, the chemistry of what goes into your body, and how the outside world looks at you, how it treats you. Jude calls herself "Schizophrenian", feeling as many do, the sting of the "schizophrenic" tag. It could go back to Adam's naming the animals, notably the one he called woman.

We find Jude's womanhood emerging in her story, first in her mad flight from her mother and father, later in the continuing love story with George where they become "Jeordy", and culminating in the arrival, growth and blossoming of their daughter Amanda.

Reading this is not easy. Schizophrenese is a language replete with word-play, puns, neologisms, alliteration, strange associations and tangential flow like Muhammed Ali's boxing to "float like a butterfly, sting like a bee'. No accident that one of the main characters here is the rock star Sting. Fans of the later James Joyce might feel at home with it.. The rest of us will find it hard to follow at first but then - if you can bear with it - find yourself entering that world and then into Jude's life as it unfolds. Never mind that it jerks you back and forth in time. Enjoy the story!

Dr Guy Mersereau MD.

Disclaimer:

Although the general consensus is that people who have Schizophrenia are lagging in word power, commonly called poverty of speech, for some reason I, myself, have no problem in expression in this manner. (Writing) My words are bound to wax cryptic. Typing my personal biography consequently is easy. If it is hard to adjust from hearing my spartan verbal word power, to a written account, which is much more confusing to those expecting simplicity, please press on and hopefully you all can recover from too MUCH information. Good Luck, and enjoy.

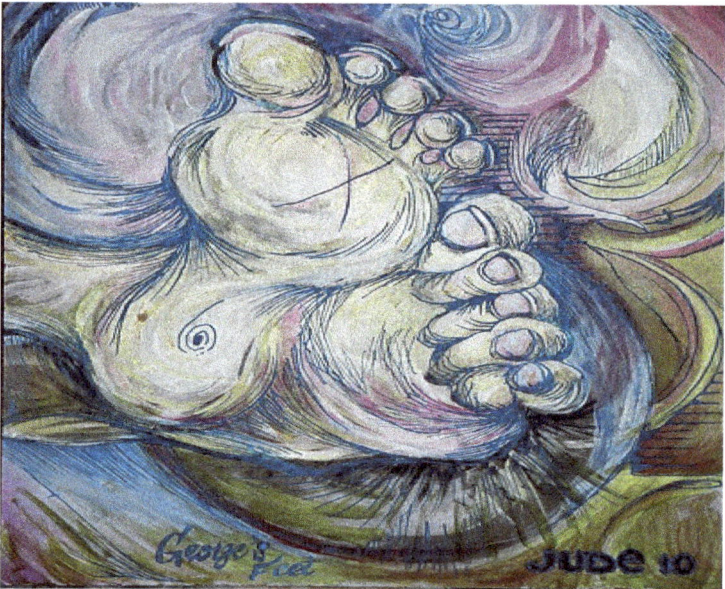

"How Beautiful are the feet of
those who bring good news"

Author's Forward

The Life of a Professional Schizophrenian

So I've been asked to elaborate on Schizophrenia and those waxing Schizophrenian. Keep in mind that this illness can be worldwide in scope whilst remaining comfy in somebody's compact personal brain. A city within itself. Those who have been granted this unfortunate citizenship are members of an elite yet most misunderstood club in their cranium. This particular metropolis is uniformly a run-down unkempt ghetto with unseen stagnant thought poverty. Even if a schizophrenian is adept at expression, the echo sounds like "poor me" instead of "understand me", and so all is interpreted as a climate of destitution. We just cannot win. Common belief concludes that we barely are able to scrape two thoughts together, and if we can...we are rendered delusional.

So what keeps us going? In one simple statement, "we exist". It's more akin to starting out by saying "I AM" and then immediately shuddering with the stark conclusion "I am SCHIZOPHRENIAN" Pretty bleak. A lifetime of poverty: poverty monetarily, poverty of diet, poverty of living arrangements, abundance of rejection, poverty of thought and conversation, regulated supplies of cigarettes (up to 90% of us smoke) But in our hearts there is soaring of the mind with stubborn rejection of this outer world's down pressing of the disabled.

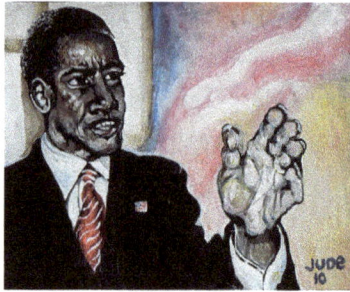

We Dream Big

We dream big. And since this wry condition cannot be pried away without medication, psychotherapy, and familial intervention, for example, since it cannot return to a happier past and still calmly reject the hopes permanently left behind, Schizophrenian becomes an elephant in the room. But there is hope for the burgeoning Schizophrenian. It does take something with the force of another elephant to clear the room of its elephant in the room(get it?) The problem is that all too often the second elephant is more resistant to vacate than the first. And so on. Perpetual perception problems. The elephant-filled room.

And what is this room?

It is a box where we exist. It is usually closed to the public until one of us citizens discovers a secret ceiling and escapes upwards for a time. When those guarding the box see this freed "clown" happy and bouncy, they frantically stifle and smother said clown down into the box. Again. Then, their particular job resumes, mindlessly cranking through life like a mass-lever round and redundantly round expecting no surprises. Alas.

Another nut gets out.

Okay. That actually is a Jack-in-the-box memory from my childhood.

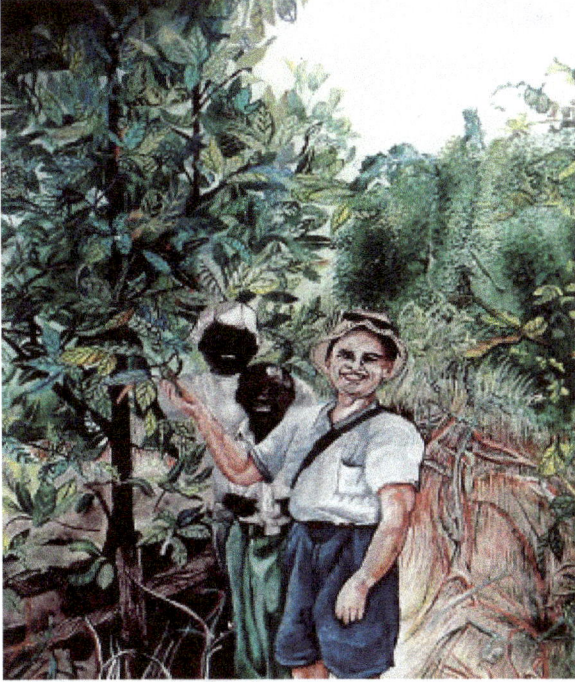

Jack OUTSIDE the Box

Here is the precise allusion. Many of us earthlings can relate to this world as containing three "worlds".

The first...that's the number-one best... is specially for the rich, overdeveloped, overweight "countries" Although some patriots are not habitually fat during their daily skinny-money marathons.

The second world, sadly enslaved by chaotic hellish communism is poor but maintains the capacity to incinerate the entire planet several times over.

The third: world music, lots of love, and no money at all in their perpetual paradise. Yay

But wait—could it be??? A fourth world? A fourth one not made up of psychiatric patients, but maybe revering them in a way. You see, the Indigenous people worldwide: the first nations...and therefore the last, hold ownership of an invisible clime, unseen by those blinded by self. No wonder it is considered magical. Anyway, these natives hold mental types as harbingers of danger, sentinels to the wind's whispers, and special with their unique gifts, even more completely unseen by other money chasers or nuclear bomb happy power mongers. But maybe observed by chance by those poor enough to relate in that third world aforementioned as poor.

And so...the Schizophrenian seen in greater accuracy by first nation ones, do really have a place to thrive and therefore are citizens by right on this orb called earth. Care to vacation in our "land?"

– Jude.
–

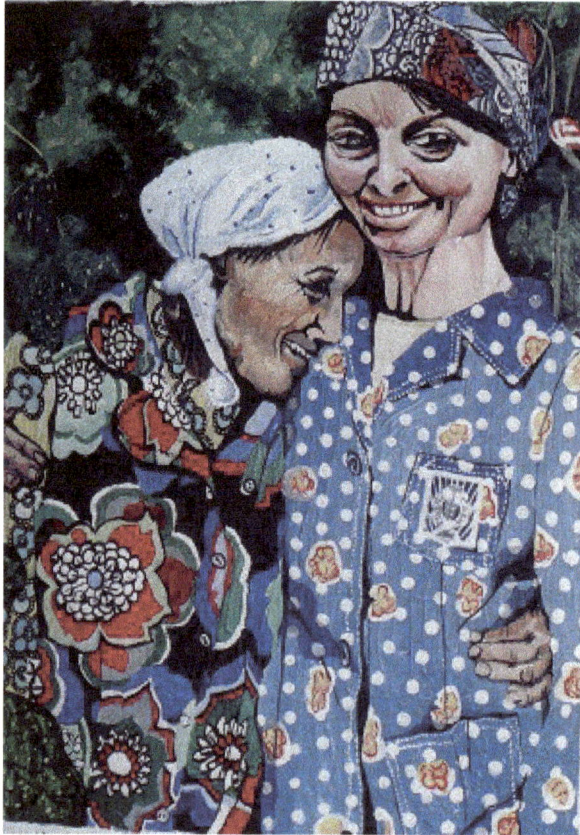

Second World Girls

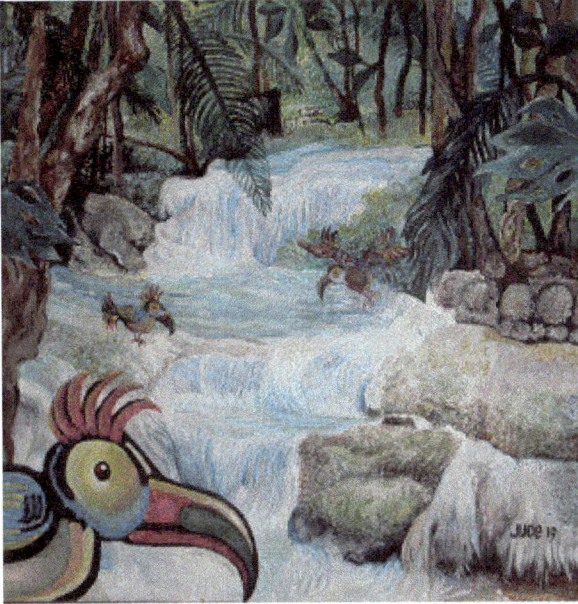

Indigenous Forest

Introduction

It takes a lot to pen a schizophrenian autobiography. Alone. Seems that the same bizarre thought patterns cannot be translated by the affected mind's mouth. What I mean is that I understand as an individual what the outside world cannot possibly anticipate or be prepared for. Like Amadeus Mozart, there are too many notes. Mine being mental notes. Mine being cloaked in my skull. So I take this risk of absolutely remaining an enigma.

It is hard to put words to symbolic events that have changed my life towards illness, it is difficult to itemize the progressive trend to insanity, it is frustrating to re-learn how to connect verbally with people who have no inkling of understanding of what I have been through, and am going through and especially to clue in to where I am taking them to: with my pen.

To disclose ideas that took years to arrive at, to release fears that have such potential energy to me alone, but could only provide a chuckle to those who think that they know any better...it is hard. In a way, by writing this book, I am saying goodbye to inaccurate thoughts, called delusions, even though these symbols meant so much to me for my temporary mental stability however fragile it may have been.

For my well-being I had to gauge the risk of giving away something precious even if it became a passing whimsical vignette whistling its way by the outsider.

I say outsider because you all reside outside of my physical skull. You have no right to peer in and only what I say can be used for conjecture by you. Unless you happen to have a CAT scan machine in your possession. So my mind-scape is solely mine, as though it is a city to inhabit by oneself solitarily. I have walked these streets alone in the presence of too many who never noticed. Like a homeless migrant loner.

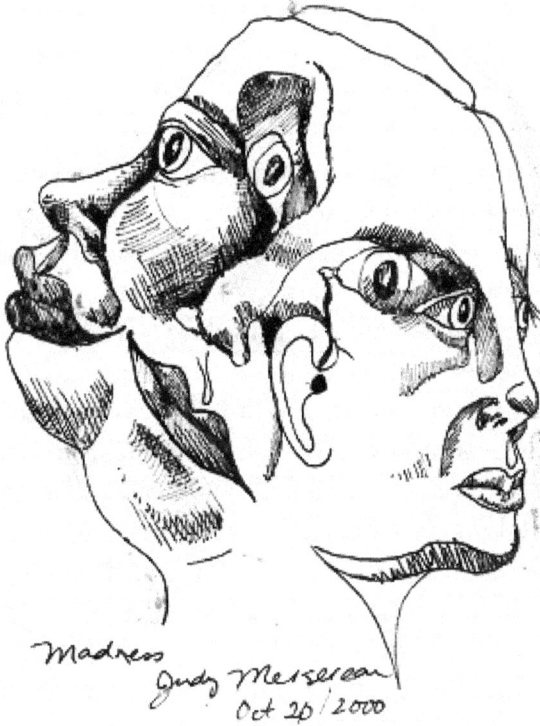

Madness Judy Messerean
Oct 20 2000

If the choice is life and demise, survival or defeat, suicide or alternatively re-hospitalization, well then the author's resultant doom-like feelings are well warranted. Expected. Anticipated. Even dreaded by inevitable self-fulfilled prophecies.

We expect the worst reaction because of the first time that we disclosed anything at all. More commonly known as our first mistake. And even to a professional (or close clone), mind you. We were given a shot of Haloperidol in our buttock and a life sentence of pain and humiliation.

Oh, and poor diet. But do they (you) understand? It is

congruent to a young monk, zealous and contrite, who can never betray their vow of silence. Ever. Even though He feels better initially to tell someone anything at all, the bad news is that he has proven himself to be a bad monk. So most people who are schizophrenian wait until they are so sick, so confused, so far gone...that they really betray their own entire personal dreamscape...treasured to them, to them alone.

Others just do not get it. From the outside world, their apathy, loss of energy, decline in hygiene, and withdrawal into oneself is similar to any young person, unlucky for the sufferer of Schizophrenia. By the time we express the symptoms of psychosis and not adolescence, it is too late to do anything but mediate and medicate.

But, sadly, this disclosure could fail to revive a modicum of empathy from most others. They reckon... Just another junk heap of gibberish. Well, it is well thought-out gibberish. Re-hashed, painstakingly rehearsed, and these ideas remain completely pure and unadulterated if kept to oneself only. Forever. Unfit for anything but Science-fiction writing of the strangest kind. This is all we are to the savvy and unmoved. Sci-fi Sages. The listeners are savvy because these professionals own the vernacular, the diagnoses, the knowledge of medications, the right to predict the level of recovery, the ultimate right to force hospitalization, and even the power to veto a simple granting to their Patient (and we are, patient by then) a basic bachelor apartment. Unmoved, because they, the professionals possess the right to go home at the end of their own special day to the house of their dreams, in a neighborhood of repute, naturally. They have no need to move, or be moved.

How, though can one person, one being, one specimen convey all that is necessary? How do you solve a problem like schizophrenia?

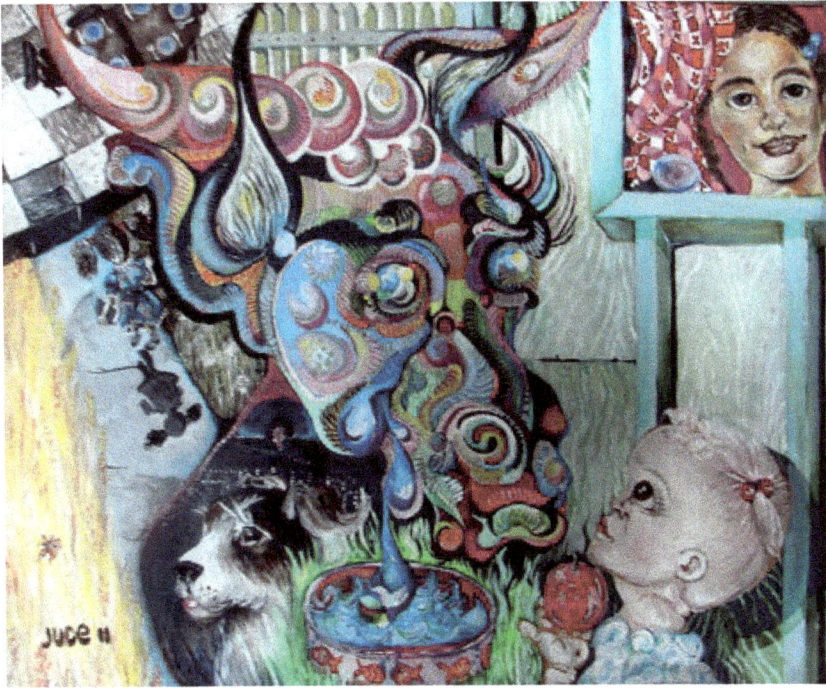

Cow

Their own desperate despair must be peeled back. That fact, wanted or not, pulled out, exposed, drawn away, and why? We, suddenly clinical cases, wonder what the point would be to a disparate, lifeless, crass world of uncaring clinicians, unshaken and overtly unmoved ones, unless they wish to be moved to a better neighborhood, perhaps? Why should we? My husband of over 31 years to this date, was once informed by his case manager that she would be leaving him behind since she had found a better job. Nice. It may be a job, and may even be work to some, but it is our LIFE.

Would it help to slow down the anticipation of what to call us, to decelerate my own explanation of the Schizophrenian experience, in particular, what group to assign us to, what level of pain to prescribe for, and at what speed of experiential guessing of our illness progression? (Prognosis)

Glean the meaning of someone's penned-out pain. This is

painful. This stuff is real on the skull interior.   Sadly only symbolic to the observer, without possessing the inside track of inner insight of the illusory.   It is lost in the translation.   We have the conundrum, you have the solutions, and never the two shall meet. Now I ask all of you...could this desert I personally travel, with my footprints disappearing soon after being trod, could this deserted city at midday, this psyche ward of silence and stillness be the exact same allegory for all, symbolically, experiencing their own personal breakdown?

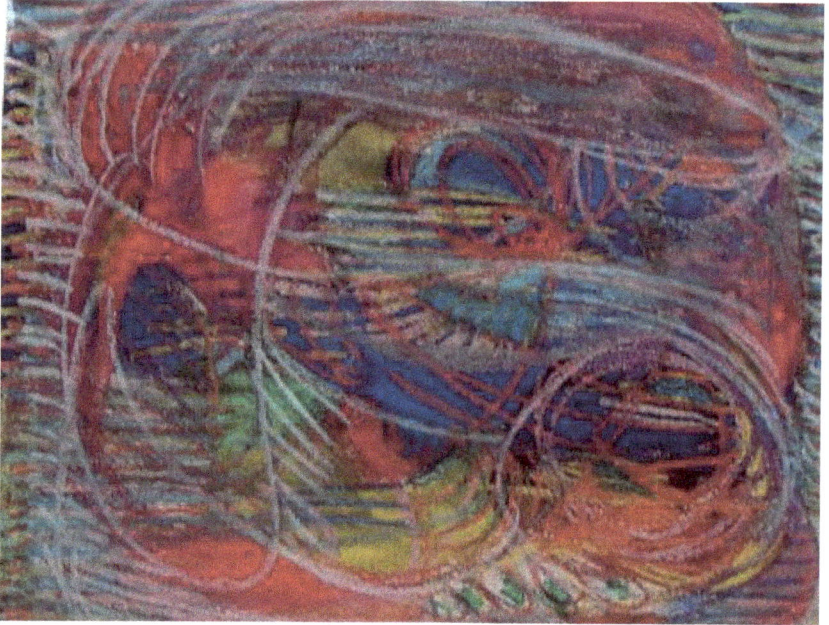

Frenetic Forest

Maybe regardless of all differences of experience "our"myriad of mentalities are the same biochemically, and hence merely a physical illness?? Or rather that every psych-patient executes the same story to all witnesses, educated or not, prepared or newly hired, Hardened or simply needing the first coffee of their day... because the Schizophrenian story needs to be heard by all, because we all boast the oddly similar deductions, similar cryptic scenarios. We are all human.

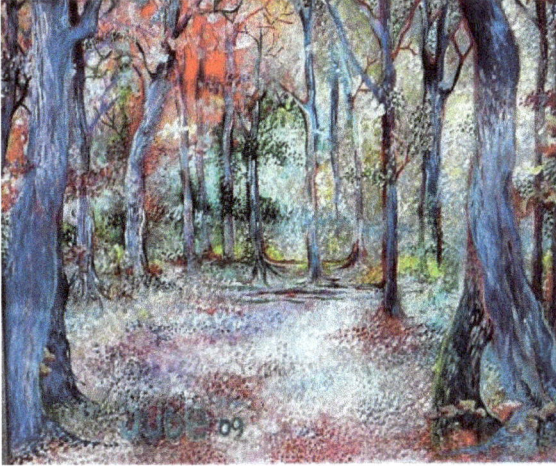

Forest Restored

And to brush off another simply due to their appearance, behavior, or lack of proper vociferating of their unique neural conclusions is a loss of precious human connection.

To ascribe to their own unique cranial configurations some respect, regardless of either being diagnosed already, or having lucidity (luckily) reassured? Okay. How about this? We all, upon our diagnosis...or life sentence...the difference is subtle... think we've reached the most perfect level. Our own synaptic state of enlightenment. Neural nirvana. Echoed in our

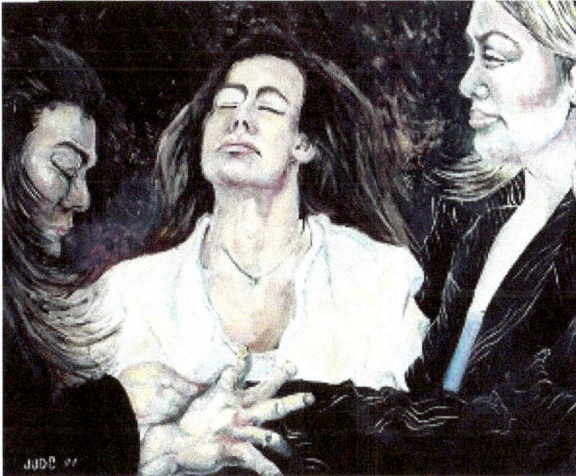

choice of subject matter and theme and scenario. Your ignorance of this is our bliss.

Let me help you all with this. Let's put a bookmark right here so that I can explain the explanation. There is no need to be a psychic. Although psychics have a field day with us gullible suggestible types, until we get too bizarre even for a mind-reader-imposter to comprehend. They seem to know us like an open book initially. They can read our minds. Until we get down to the nitty gritty. So, having been rejected by a few psychics and their fear, I have resorted to tedious typing out of what THEY even recoiled away from. To create a good "read" one should be expected to, encouraged to, divulge seeds of thought...whether authentic or not.

St. Paul wrote,"Am I really insane? It is for God's sake. Or am I sane? It is for your sake". The risk of being caught in ERROR(?) after establishing trust with someone gifted in insight and freak them out with your mind wide-open—leads to panicked fear, gargantuan both sides. Awaiting criticism from droves of all-seeing priceless minds to see all...it is . No simple ego, no matter how big; denial, no matter how consolidated; or delusion no matter how devious can negate this embarrassing thought that what the weirdo in question has decided to do is basically inspire a free-for-all for those devoid of mental malaise; mental illness. Although the fear of being discovered is far more powerful than any so-called mind-reader's scrutiny and their ability to "read minds." Curious?

People laugh. And it stings. Okay, maybe they cower away, also.

I was initially overjoyed to share my various delusions and illustrious deductions; consequently my opinions about...you know... rape, brain-damage, loss of social contacts, I learned very quickly to shut-up and smile. Whilst the Resident Psychiatrist gobbled multitudinous symptoms and proceeded to sight his own guaranteed wonderful private practice on the near horizon. (so, grin and bear it). Oh, and one must be patient and wait for hours to receive an "audience" with a psychiatrist. As though the entire world does not hear your thoughts, anyway.

Any generic autobiography writer writes and reveals their thought up peculiarities to make the book interesting no doubt. For I, to disclose to my judging public, any of an assortment of fallacies, eclectic abnormalities, or pertinent mental adventures with significant abandon, is scary. Being left unrestrained (remember straight-jackets?) is scary.

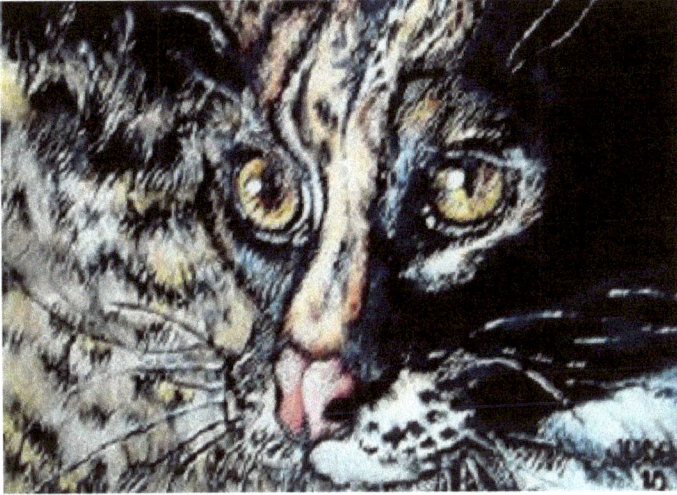

Very scary. But I have to. I must. It seems that I am quite able to vociferate this yukky stuff. I've discovered the fact that if you starve a weed, it will die. And if you broadcast openly your secret sensibilities, ignoring personal paranoia, well, you're getting somewhere! "YOUR SECRETS KEEP YOU SICK" is a popular adage, adeptly announced by those in recovery, regardless of their success with sanity (or reasonable facsimile). We all learn to confess our stuff. But why is there so little, so far, in our life-account that talks about events or real life occurrences? Because our lives became an inner event and our breakdown recurs to us daily, anew. New nuances. Fresh newness to face up and 'fess up. We are so busy observing our spectrum of symptoms that we do not see the rainbows all around, designed to distract.

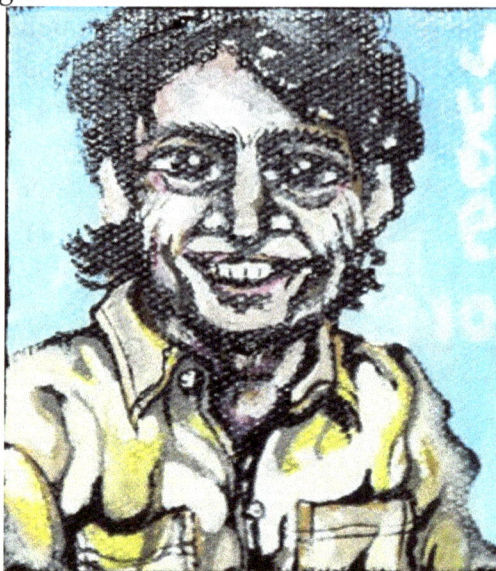

Georgie

My husband, George, and I decided to live our lives anyway, in spite of any symptom or side-effect. That meant that sometimes we were... ...caught in the world between sanity and Hell, for lack of a worse word. So. Why? Why should one gregarious girl with her cleverly cornered Schizophrenia and her stone-cold solution to psychosis shake the cryptic corner-stone of Psychiatry itself? The professionals already know that their practice of suspicious-teeth- pulling is an alternate complementary vocation. Without the dental tools. Why should any one solitary Psychiatrist become curious of such a patient...and more importantly, why would I become such a curious patient? Pardon the cryptic English.

-why not?-

Philosophy aside. Thoughts wind and meander from synapse to beleaguered synapse in the brain of the insane. These synapses are slippery. As soon as one singular idea has been isolated, identified as erroneous, although original in content as it may be, the next synapse is ready to adopt all the information, leaving this idea undetected...not pinpointed, for now. Neural prowess is in the excess. We grow clever to protect the innocence. This brain has learned to be coy with frustrated counsellors' "convincing skills"   Logical thought initially initiated from outside and genuinely attempted to graft onto this injured brain, renders itself non-effectual...at first. Being doped up in a Dopamine deterrent medication makes us adopt zombie-like attributes, and then the subsequent worldwide universal rejection strengthens and consolidates confused "idea" cells (ironically called receptors) as we try and try again to explain outward with our reaching out that we are misunderstood. That fact is noted as a misconception, another delusion. Ironic and logically impossible. Shouldn't one's statement of realization that they are different be considered as a harbinger of turning the corner? Reviving of self?

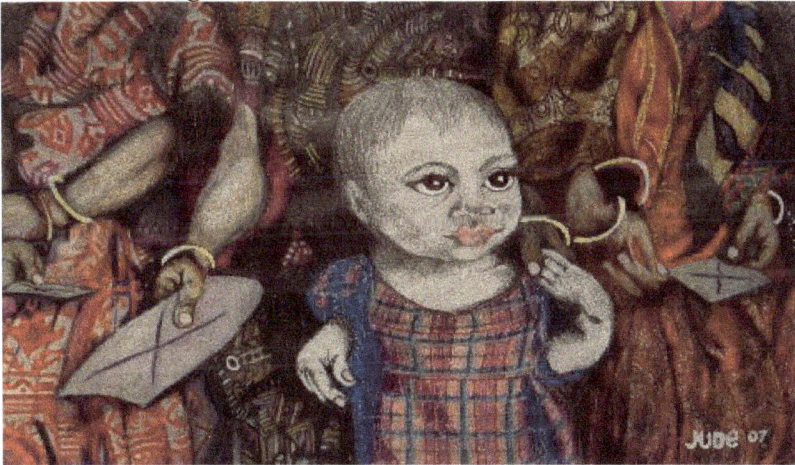

"A-Mandatory- Assimilation"

Since the illness emanates outward from an unknown source inside, that is foreign to consciousness, these thoughts of liberation from normalcy are oddly original to the untrained eye of...the otherwise normal. We all have a hidden subconsciousness; but just because yours is still unconscious does not make you BETTER, pardon the pun.

To maintain the deluded stance is to deploy a biological defense mechanism usually initiated at the first question of psychotherapy..."Do you hear voices?" Clever. This installs a springboard to recovery. The thoughts go like this...once one realizes that voices are known to this abruptly caring soul. One then panics, "How does she know I hear voices?" "Maybe I should say they are not my voices" "Maybe she can hear the voices!" "Perhaps the whole world is listening." "I've been found out!" --We deny everything. The experiment is a resounding success as the response is tantamount to self-criticism, along with self-preservation instincts deployed. The inner dialogue is re-established, reversing psychosis one brain cell at a time. One then decides, and it is a sliding scale, just what level of acceptance they will exercise...today. Thinking that I was being clever I lied about what my voices were saying, in order to remain private, to protect my accumulation of deviance. Very valuable voices.

Only personal hardship such as working at a fast food conglomerate forever, or unneeded reduction of medication or disintegrated support where trusted ones refuse to hear anymore about YOUR stressors, since you are not the only one, after all...only some life experiences can cause relapse. Well, we kind of...are the only ones. So then, the thought that those meds are making you sick(?) and so reducing your dosage will help(?)...does not help. Such stunts like these will further feed any (or many) episode of mental breakdowns. So medication and case management along with periodic sessions with which to appease your Psychiatrist... gets the job done. And also, please stay away from the marijuana. But wait. There is more. In my personal bumper crop of crazies, our generation, born with the advent of psych meds that ran head-to-head with experimental street drugs as to which were more popular, the medications were inferior. But they improved to become today's treatments.

And although the errant mental makeup had been eventually ceased and addressed, with old-fashioned drugs, it was normal to take years to find one's way out of the crazed maze. One actually would seem to be getting worse in their recovery. As though we were better off psychotic and off antipsychotic medication. But such a revelation warrants no discontinuation of medication. Ever. What follows in this book is my attempt to illustrate. So let us start with an illustration...a glass

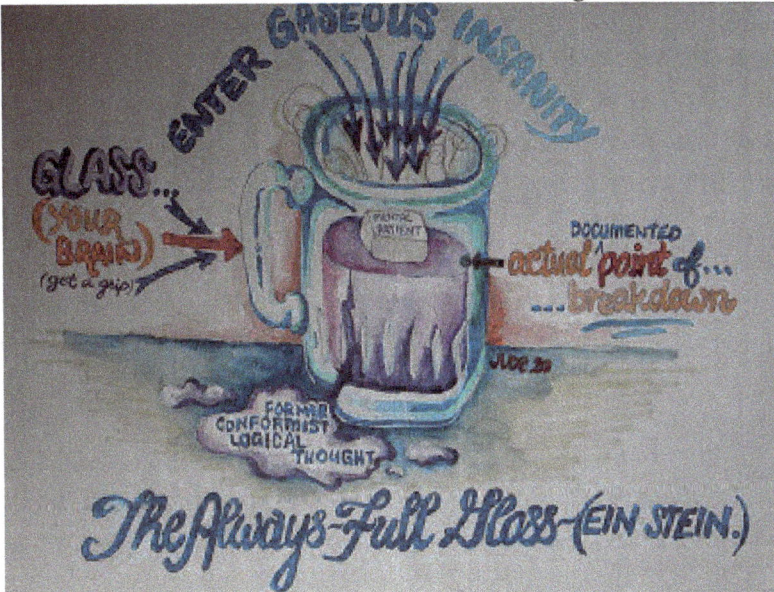

The Always-Full Glass (EIN STEIN.)

Moving progressively, yay, I will brave a betrayal of a novel idea. Say that I am better and have an angle on analogies about illness. Droves of symbolism. Say mental-like ones. With the death of free flying fantasy and the inevitable inception of self examination, the reassurance of resurgence of WELL thoughts is welcomed with relief. By everybody. Soon, the affected individual gets the hang of it. Victims of variant ventures, vast and invisible, introspective and intense, adopt a sense of post-psychosis compromise. We still remember our former state, but eventually, opt for recovery, if we are capable, and honest with all, especially our own selves. Now, that is not so crazy; it is healthy. Habitual wellness. Although laborious for patient and professional throughout the experience.

So, here comes the fun part. We all sheepishly see the glass as half-full or half-empty, do we not? Well, what if, observing the totality of experiences everywhere, all around us, worldwide, overflowing with abandon, like the Psalmist's Psalm says,"My cup runneth over.", we realize that that glass is ALWAYS full? All admit hopefulness or nemesis gladly. We choose, playfully one or the other. Air or liquid. Deep or pie-in-the-sky. Sane or insane. Nonetheless, we all are residing somewhere in this glass, (remember skulls?), with our insupportable findings from fantasy unfulfilled or our non-sympathetic judgments on mental pathology, whether good or faltering, on any level or fullness of findings. Make sense? Maybe to somebody, I can guarantee.

Even the cognitive giants can engender erroneous conclusions, however minute to them. These grandiose guesses bubble over into the forbidden higher airiness of inspiration. But basically, the norm chooses to reside at the glass-bottom. Here the dense, shape-conforming glass inhabitants huddle at the glass's bottom- half, like water, hanging out in safety and, at least not possessing unmentionable and stinky gaseousness, and thinking like those glass-top explorers, with their inert character and characteristic creative flatulence. Artsy fartsy to the limit. All is well for both sides of sanity with a succinct line of delineation. That is right, between the two—the heights of logic bottom up, and the edge of breakdown in a downward spiral-effect...both drawn at a very fine line, exactly at the halfway level of the glass. What a coincidence! They say there is a fine line between genius and insanity.

see illustration   And then there are the borderline cases of mental illness (wellness?).

Now, people, if said glass affords a crack, oh never!   Fissure in its foundation,   humanity! Upwards   towards   the cusp of sanity/insanity, oh no! Whatever shall we do? This lovely NORMAL liquid   escapes   as   it bottoms out, and then the

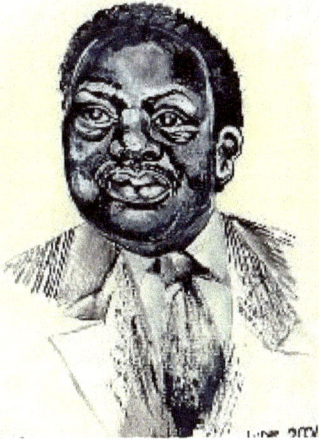

Genius

freed radical thought invades the normal domain.   Enter breakdown. The glass is your mind. (see illustration) What is left is a bunch of nonsensical interpretations of the territory formerly- and covertly, suppressed by the water-dwellers symbolic anomalies and unresolved conflicts... hidden junk. These problems, once been swept under the rug,,, now find the selfsame rug pulled out from under themselves. Hence mental illness.

This rug junk cannot be explained with the insufficient vernacular of some top of the glass one, plunging towards the cracked bottom of a glass. Then medication can fill such a crack, and with psychological watering cans, refilling that glass some new seeds of sanity can grow. Basic stuff, no?

So, can something so non-substantial as gas, lacking lead-like protection (from a glass formally half- filled with water), unearth formerly buried symbolism, those that afford delusion? Confusion? Erroneous psychosis? When it is housed in one's personal broken-down brain it leaks reality away like a nuclear accident, airing the radioactive side of notion as refreshing as a breeze of fresh "err".

Just some thought fodder for your fancy.

Jude

MADNESS

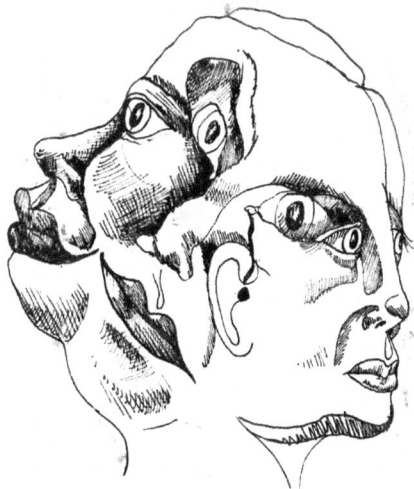

Book One

Chapter One

"Where do we go? Where do we go, now?"
-Guns "n" ro*ses*

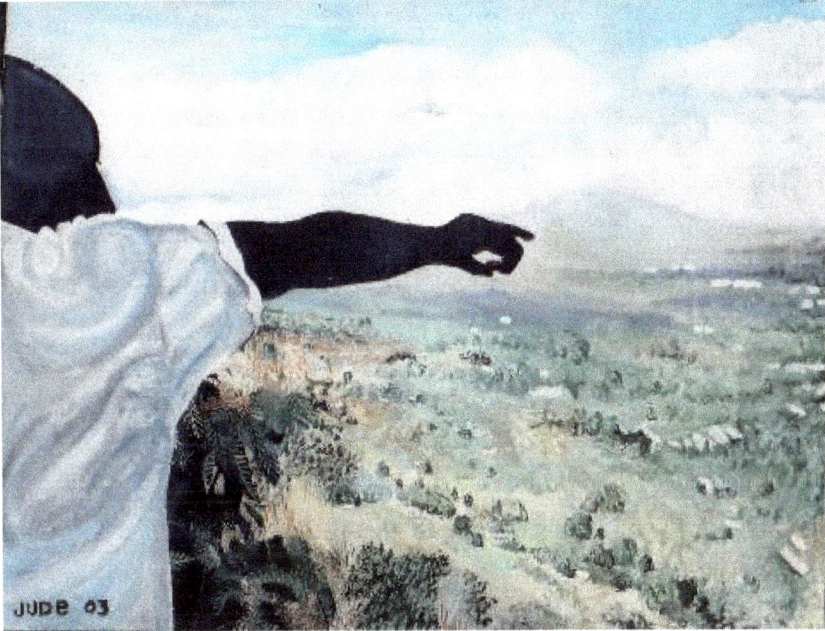

Datwehso

When presented with the carefully coaxed cluster of cells in the cranium in question, of which my own thoughts call home, the answer to this is mutually exclusive. Everywhere AND nowhere. NOW is the key. NOW is the answer. Everything is in the present. It is an internal inferno burning right now.

The Psalmist David wrote: "Where can I go from Your presence, LORD...If I make my bed in Hell, You are there"-139, vs. 8

How about the recent Global pandemic which hastened

everybody's wilderness sojourn whether with or without a fever and diarrhea? Having to face oneself directly as the days blend together into one relentless opera of the redundant absurd variety is parallel to an average mental breakdown without the threat of concrete lungs ending all things abruptly. Premature death for mental types takes time...of which we afford in unified accord

Many   many   years   of   mediocre

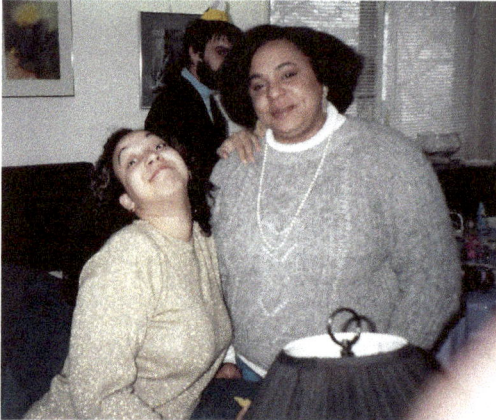

Big Sis Little Sis

diet and excessive ciggys accompanied with lax exercising regimes and an imposed lesser potential for success in any particular echelon of life takes a serious toll on our bodies...and our own unique productive thoughts lag on from a deceptively defective mind.(really?)

Everybody that has had a six month or so stay at their friendly neighborhood psych ward knows intimately the leagues of useless symptoms, endless symptoms, medically submerged symptoms. They sadly lack buoyancy and neither can they tread water. So as we are wont to remain delusional we pace the ward floor wistfully or in a listless lament-laden dance. There is no more above water existence. Just "reality"...bare and stripped down to a non- fluid necessity.(see the illustration again) We float like an ice-cube at the sanity or insanity cusp.

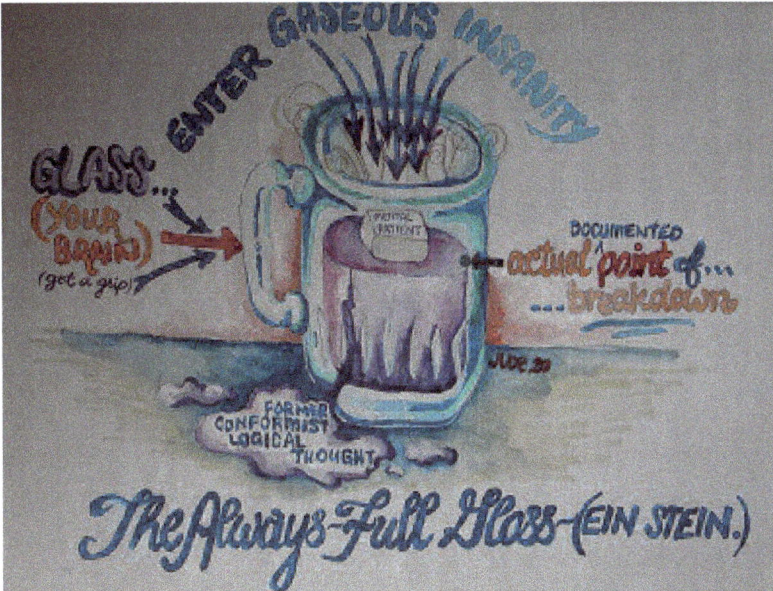

The Always-Full Glass (EIN STEIN.)

There is still ultimately the initial agitation, evidence of remaining brain activity. But these unfortunate souls still have no point of logic where it meets the edge of sanity. They have bottomed-out. EVERY single thing is conscious with no "liquid" to buffer the rougher stuff into subconscious submission. There are some things we just do not need to remember or relive. But we do, anyway. The scope of these two reality extremes are as tantamount as guns and roses are in symbolism. So, I echo and elaborate, elucidate and concur...where DO we go? Obviously we have been there already and it seems we are stuck. Highly educated types dare not initiate any observation of something so unseen and merely guess at the unexpressed...so invisible. It is called an ice-cube at the bottom of a glass, people!

Case in point:

Life...was dull...I had...been...having trouble getting...past...time elapsed...chronicling it. So...since I had...already started smok...ing...(i.e., I had turned 18)...cigarettes...began to...document those time passages in...greater accuracy. Once the lit butt singed my flannel pajama leg as I lounged on the couch in that room with a television and a sofa and a chesterfield… and began to burn the skin on my thigh, I knew that approximately six minutes had elapsed which proved I was not stuck. It was now 1:17 p.m. Time for another cigarette or I will get stuck. Unbeknownst to the nurses on their rounds I was doing rather well in my polka-dotted pants.

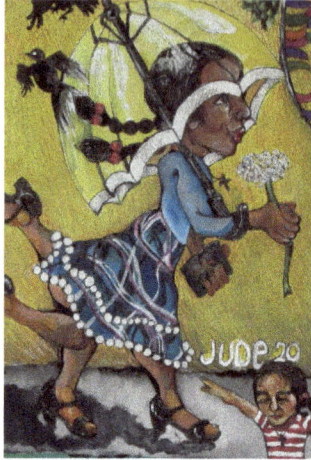

Running Real Fast

Flash forward: My dad, while experiencing his own final decline called Dementia was once found in the mid-nighttime running frantically back to bed from the bathroom. Mom inquired, "Why are you running?" My dad replied in all honesty, "So that my brains won't fall out before I get to bed!" Childlike insight to the end.

So, what was precisely that which I repeatedly got stuck IN? In the immediate parsec of time(to pinpoint the origin of psychosis perfectly) let's say that one solitary brain cell decides to deviate from normalcy and take a "dive" for the benefit of the leftover gray masses. It matters. Let us then say that some semblance of a synergic synaptic ripple seduces weak neighborhood dwelling cells surrounding this deviant dot. One cell, then three. Then thirteen in exponential multiplicity. Now, the once healthy laptop of lucidity has a virus. Let's say, now that these curious cells create an unpleasant stir biochemically and the one young skull housing this personal neural abnormality automatically seeks a solution, a satisfactory remedy. A bookmark for respite from a lifetime of rampant dreamscapes.

Does she reach out? Laughter...maybe fear. Or does she keep it secret, accelerating illness in the waning water level below the former half-full glass-line? The dilemma remains that anyone with the gift of sight can see into this cracked glass; or with the gift of insight, can detect desperate behavior, or often complete stillness, coming from a broken brain. The condition festers until someone inevitably discovers a water-less cracked glass all forlorn and disabled.(see the illustration).

Diet? One could become a macrobiotic vegan vegetarian and still reap the grim reality of a virtual vegetative state. Regardless. Seriously.

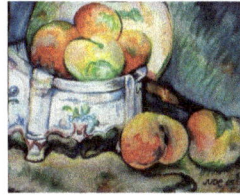

Vitamins? Vital to those not YET affected. Sadly, late-acting for the slowly motivated psych-ward dweller's demands.

Drugs?(of the street variety) Fast-track to the hospital. Sorry.

And therefore these stress susceptible cells inaugurate an unprecedented scenario where the inner and outer worlds are at odds. Typical teen, right? But with Schizophrenia, "reality" is the odd-one-out. And there renders no solution logistically. The same brain that can interpret its mental malady is hampered with disarmed logic ammunition stores. Thought-speech-insight-solution chains of thought-speech-insight-solutions. Medication intervention gives the sufferer a chance to catch their breath neurologically and start from a "better" framework. The word "better" has never been so apropos, so the recovering one surmises. But let us dig deeper in the dirt, since it is so sinking to the one who...sinks.

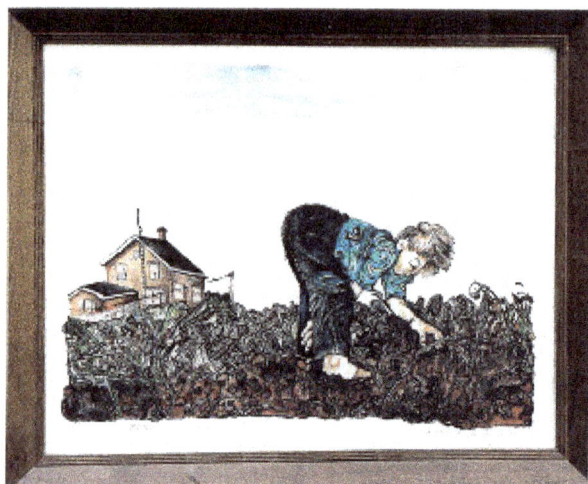

Digging in the Dirt

Chapter Two: Enter Dopamine!

Firstly, to the families and friends, please never say "they are no DOPE-of-MINE!" We need you more now than ever, us unlucky flunkies. We are not dopes and we long to have a fixed up family, like it was in times past. All families have someone with mental concerns. In fact, one in four suffer, whether thought disruptions, or mood misconduct, from hoarding, to

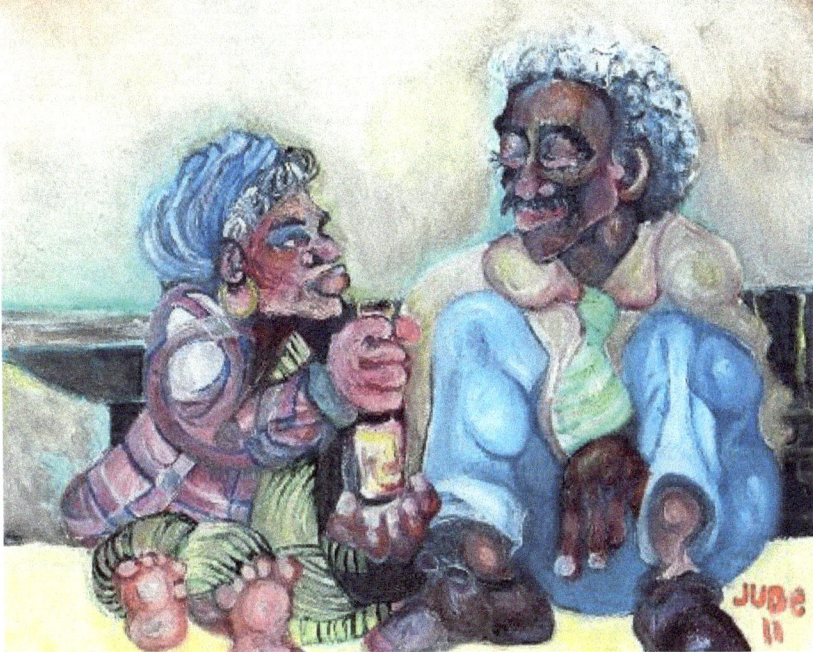

"Care for some wine?"

drinking to whatever comes out of the hat. So how do we get stuck, and why is the goal always complete recovery and not, at least at first, reconciliation? Contemplative inventory decisions? Taking a deliberate self-pointed inventory. Let's see...   One gets stuck with too much stucco as they simply study ceilings. In remotely different wording, a young mind cannot realize the heights it has apparently achieved, and comprehend that it is truly "sick" so if that mind ever cares to reside in the established world again, then that the ensuing medication "ceiling" is meant for convalescent contemplation and coaxed cognitive climbing of a lesser sort. It is all about levels. We all want to reach Heaven, but some are a little too impatiently clever in their decision to soar to the heights. There is a reason that gravity exists. To keep us in the real world that we all are wont to reject. We are all needed in this mess called Earth. Christians explain that we are both SAINT and SINNER while sojourning in this world. Those two realities are cohabitating. Then MEDIcation can MEDIate in the marriage of sanity and insanity... formerly glass-crushing attitudes. Once a much more realistic height- goal is made, a new expectation, a lesser level, the newly disabled young adult ponders their lowered ceiling, gradually getting used to the new, mundane, muted thoughts. The patient patient eyes all the nuances on their novel and less-expectant thought-blocked ceiling which others can call stucco. Soon, staccato strings of sensible sentences are summoned from their subconscious. They are getting better, these young ones.

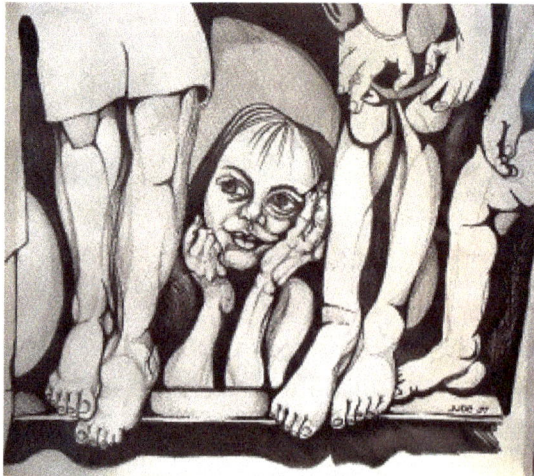

Resilience

How does this happen? A medicated, and newly adjusted point of sanity, much lower in expectation, (and lower in the glass on that wonderful philosophical illustration) can aid a recovery although slow in progress. This ceiling produces the most beautifully stubborn patterns of outcomes in hopes of reviving frustrated delusional dregs which linger at the glass bottom. Once the hospital's guest sojourner acknowledges their situation and its non-spacey finality they can now see that the ozone is the limit and reality below is where it is to be. So, after about half a year of studying stucco ceilings, someone special is primed for discharge.

Why do the psychiatrists put a cap on creativity, other than the fact that psychologists lack the credentials themselves? And why does this involve so much stucco ceilings? What about popcorn ceilings, for example? They encourage the organization of each single explosive kernel of thought...blocked or not. Most newly crazy ones are granted popcorn ceilings, or rather, newer medications, like Clozapine, which has kept me out of the hospital for more than 25 years. Nonetheless, once a new reality-recruit is ready for living outside the ward, they are granted a disability pension and shuffled off to a nice second-level lodging home.

If only boarding houses painted skies and clouds on their ceilings, maybe one would have hope. But the situation inside a second level lodging home provokes frustration and anger and causes one to question the psychotic life left behind as the "problem" after all. Medication is restrictive and stifling and zombie producing and embarrasses the heck out of some zombie not aware that "psychiatric" means strange, to ordinary people. I use the word "ordinary" because so-called superiors have long ago given up on productive thought. Not a nanosecond of originality. So they really cannot afford an extra cigarette to someone who will only use it for an attempt to reach pot-like heights, once attained long ago, and forever hampered by the same medicine that makes them...zombies. Any one of us who smoke in memory of marijuana imagine we possess the ability to

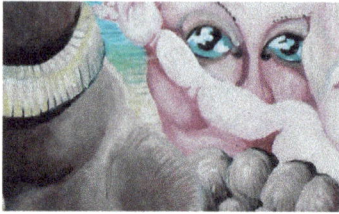

change tobacco to ganja at will. These others, lovely intellectual flunkies, need their OWN cigarettes for their timed cigarette breaks where they spew expert sarcastic remarks about their wizened world and avoid those false, fat freaks who huddle downtown and lurk at the portal of every doughnut shop. Needing a coffee. Needing a cigarette to simply stay awake. Don't these "rich" ones realize that it is better to give? Receptors react favorably to the nicotine 'HIT' in the schizophrenian frontal lobe… the part of the brain needed for higher thought and executive decisions...no wonder we are called professional schizophrenics. Our occupation is annoying to otherwise happy office slaves, whose primary care is to fit TWO cigarettes and one medium coffee into a scheduled work break. Stucco ceilings: Stopping psychosis.

Some never adopt the hovering limits imposed in order to re-establish sanity. The creative gene never devolves into the ordinary one. We do not see the need to abandon the Mountain-top experience as we descend, medicated, to the valley below. Meds restore logic only, and these lucky few recovered ones

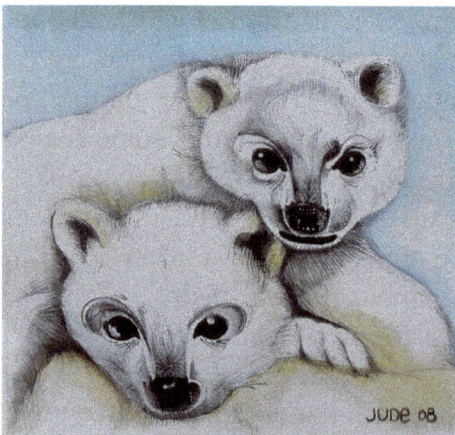

retain their memories of grandeur and fresh air at altitudes above. Somehow, upon total recovery, the world is in awe of some nut's Sistine Chapel where the rest remained stuck at stucco.

These recovered ones can make the best psychiatrists although most of the actual

JUDE 08

Bi-Polar

36

successful graduates sell out for mere stucco solutions. Pardon my anger, if detected. I myself discovered that I was one of the "Lucky 15%" from a resident Orthopedic Surgeon—to which I dutifully chimed that the rate of Schizophrenia was only one in one hundred people. To which he happily revealed that the new statistic was that a full 15% of people suffering schizophrenia recovered COMPLETELY. Oh, Happy Day! So I am NOT crazy. Well.

Shall we? Going on...how did we all arrive there, in our castles in the air, clouds 'n' all? While I, myself, was handling High School as a stable genius, my illness barged into the classroom and took a quick look at those sitting, studying; it pitched a tent and decided to become... a squatter. Nobody saw this event. Like all squatters are...my psychosis went unnoticed. As long as there were educational parameters, rules that I could still mimic conformity to and with, my transient thoughts went on to grow, prodding further deviance. I was getting sick, and no-one noticed since my overt creativity was being watched and all bets were on what I should become. My mental mutation maintained anonymity, standing undetected. Residual brilliance. When I visited the Guidance Counselor in mid grade twelve, I was told that my grades were well within my dream of being a Psychiatrist (You heard it here), but would I rather, a Psychologist? I answered, "Whichever is more difficult".

For example, and I am being ridiculous, people, in math class, we were fed sine and cosine...I was tangential, writing over and over "He's out of my life", a song written in a similar manner by Michael Jackson, a famous pop star of the time. French. I decided to instill an evolved grammatical system in a creative presentation, hoping to mend Canada's language barriers, but instead delivered a risky esoteric schizophrenic skit. My teacher immediately retorted, "bizarre" (which means "bizarre" in English.) In English class, I breezed into the final exam with 93% and managed...to fail the final examination.

So much for school.

Did I mention the adventure of summer school? For three summers in a row, I courageously attended morning classes for the interim months of summer,. in order to receive extra courses, in order to graduate early. This means if you know your math, that I had no educational break for approximately four years. When I was still fifteen, there was only one subject lacking to make a full high school diploma. I took a "victory lap"

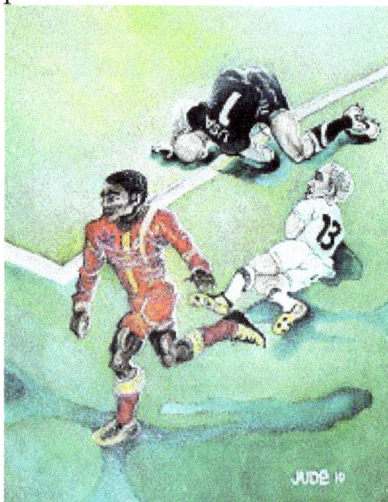

Ghana beats the 'States

For my second year of grade twelve I managed to graduate with a healthy 87% average, with about 37 credits. (only approximately 28 courses were needed.) Maybe I burned out? Most of the extra credits were from art courses, my chosen field, so I really didn't mind. After graduating, there was the Graduate Prom. About ten guys asked me to accompany them, so to be fair I went alone. Still I took one last course, Chemistry to complete the prerequisites for an eventual Physician's curriculum. It was the summer of 1983. I was slipping. By the end of the summer I knew that carbon-14 was dangerous and if someone announced that I was to "consider them gone", I was not to oppose such eloquence by adding, "You can't say that".

That was the summer which was dominated by Summers

and Copeland and Sumner, sadly for me. I would stray into the school library on my break from summer school studies to discover more and more mentally cryptic allusions...and it did not matter which book I took off the shelves...they all had secret meanings within the paragraphs, meant for me alone. I had one lifeline...a girl named Trudy, who wore her cheerleading sweater on the inaugural day of twelfth year chemistry summer school, coincidentally in sync with my sporting off the same, from my high school, with my own name of course. So I bellowed instantaneously, "Hey, we could be best friends...Trudy and Judy!!!" But this was not the nineteen-fifties, and my youthfulness was showing.

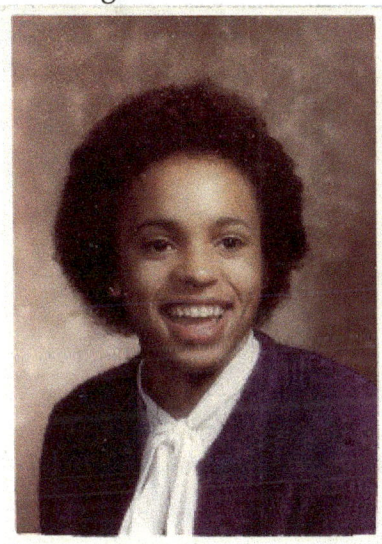

Trudy glared. In the following weeks, she would explain that she needed one last credit to finish High School, in order to go on into her profession of choice, acting. Therefore, she needed a nose-job since she suffered a nose-first collision with a truck and was going to go on as an actress. She also had an 'in' with a backstage pass to the Police Picnic on August 3rd, in Toronto. Not knowing the implications of possessing one last friendship in the real world, I waxed frenetic in true mad style, leaving my own novel biochemical trail. I managed to hang on for three days until Trudy returned from her midweek luncheon, all of three days, with the hottest band in the world. She related to her meeting Sting and his reciprocal smiling, immediate. That was the limit—I immediately had a 'vision' that was imperative to relate to Sting in person...but I was beginning to realize that Trudy truly was not my best friend. She was her own. How could all of these coincidences happen in succession that summer? Looking back I leave it alone as just some synchronistic magic somewhere betwixt sanity and...losing it all.

And I truly did.

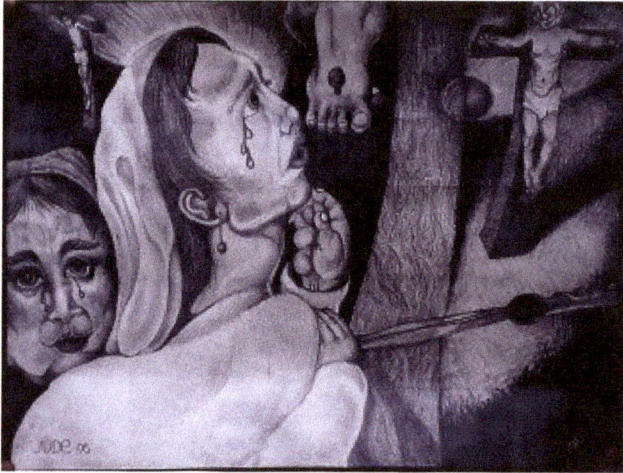

No greater Sorrow

Following my High School career, I careened into grade 13. This is the place where the teachers do not care any more in hopes of "smartening up" these smart ones in preparation for University. I recessed into that self-same lame-brain, crippled with little interest in real-time reality. The buzz going around the Hamilton Collegiate Institute was pot and Castaneda. The marijuana to my great Jamaican shame made me black-out for hours and hours. So, in compensation, I devoured the five existing Carlos Castaneda shamanism paperbacks. In one week. The five bound accounts of some anthropology student's hopeful furtherance into the spiritual shaman world made a subatomic inner-detonation dopamine cloud in my head. Geometry class produced a hefty 26% average. And I was trying, too. Advanced french reaped 92% so I dropped the course to concentrate on art. Makes sense?

Finally, the guidance counselors were wise to me and soon one of them arrived at my day-long Art class where I hid, drawing pictures of the eye of Sting, All day. She ranted about how I was a cop-out (no pun please), and as her pupils got more and more minute, I began to laugh. Knowing that those pupils betrayed the fact that she was afraid of this pupil. She was livid…and found an age loophole, since I had skipped grade one, once upon a time, sort of, and was therefore underage, and now my conduct could be reported to my parents.

Dad was crying, and could not deduce why I had dropped out. So I told him what I could, that I needed maybe to know what it is to fail at something. Talks and meditation ensued until all involved agreed that I would continue in Art with Drama as a minor course.

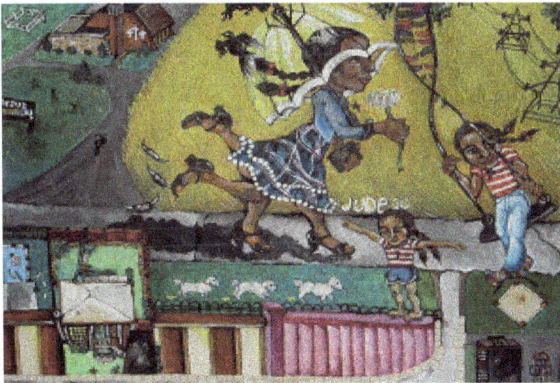

The Runaway

I had been in this former Broadway play called RUNAWAYS, an ensemble production about, runaways, and was type-cast to a degree as a drug addicted Rasta teen, who did not care anymore. My first performance, ever, on stage won me an OUTSTANDING performance award. And I was getting psychotic, too. So, in my Jude way, I dropped the Drama course and spent all my days in the art room making larger and larger eyes, with eyelashes that resembled talons and contained a myriad of increasingly-off colors. Normal brained people, even artists, usually do not paint a succession of four-feet wide eyes as their body of work. How I fared at my art college interview was a direct result of my experience in grade thirteen. I knew how to act the part, I had lots of bizarre artwork, and I had become fearless, at seventeen. I was asked to stay and wait for about an hour at the Ontario College of Art. So I did wait...finally listening to someone outside of my brain. They then brought out the good news that this girl-child had been accepted immediately to the College.

By the way, you can tell how sick one is by sizing the increasing eye size in a painting they have produced.

I WAS SICK.

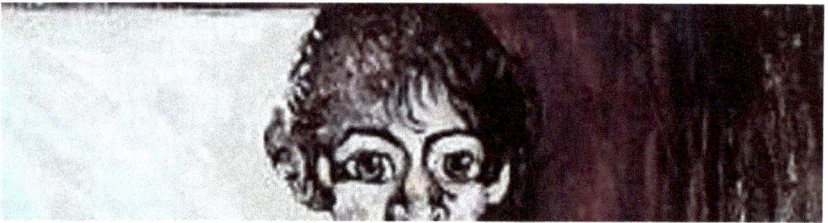

Not so "BIG" eyes

Luckily for me, my problems-unresolved, were not Religious, or Theological, or grandiose concerning God, but merely lacking comprehension of the bastardization of many people's beloved Reggae music and it's consequent compromised noble intent. I think Elvis Presley, a popular dead rock star, did the same thing, pioneering lyrical adulteration and sexual convulsing onstage for the purpose of mass adoration and money. The Beatles, a genius Sixties rock group promptly followed-suit. So when the Police enforced their regime, I, all of twelve, was unable to discern. No secret messages were needed, no anti-Jamaican sentiments, no refusal to conform to the Rastaman Vibration...just perfectly beautiful music about prostitutes, under-aged girls, inappropriate Teacher-Student liaisons, and vengeful stalking of unfaithful (I wonder why) spouses, topped the charts and conquered the hearts of an adoring unduly attentive audience. My once brilliant mind was what was affected—only. Not my spirit...NOT my soul. I tried to compute secretly, in an inward spiral that had no answer...no solution to my troubled devolution...but then, "I remembered" something special...or someone, rather. My Georgie...no-one else's. What is time, anyway, but a fabrication made by man to keep everybody hopping, when I did not get around much, anymore. So, my faith was preserved in my heart, which ultimately belonged to God and my mind was temporarily decimated with sub-standard-stuff.

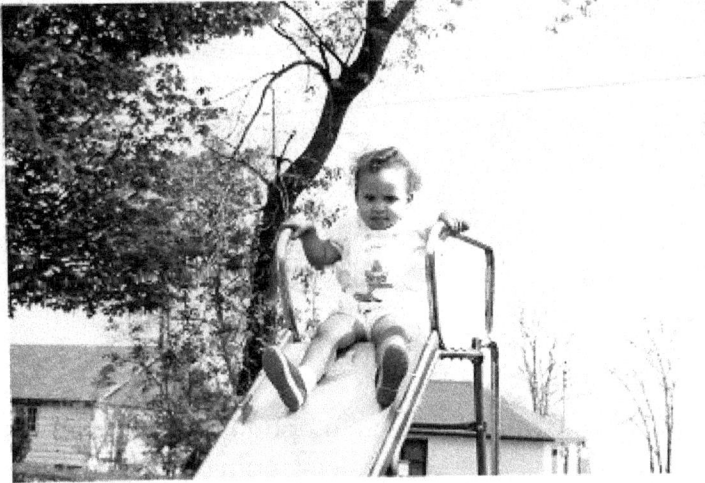

;

"You get to the bottom, you go back to the top of the slide, then you stop and you turn and you go for a ride..."
Sir Paul McCartney

My minister was right. Somewhere in my body was the real Judy, and none should lose hope over temporary situations, however dismally these times manifested themselves.

Remember...suicide is a permanent solution to a temporary problem.

So, what's Thirty-five years of constant anguish?

My Husband Georgie's Psychiatrist once remarked that he did not have time for my existential angst...and it was a good thing, since, that angst kept the edge in my life, my art, my choice of songs to perform in the Hamilton Program for Schizophrenia (HPS) Idol,

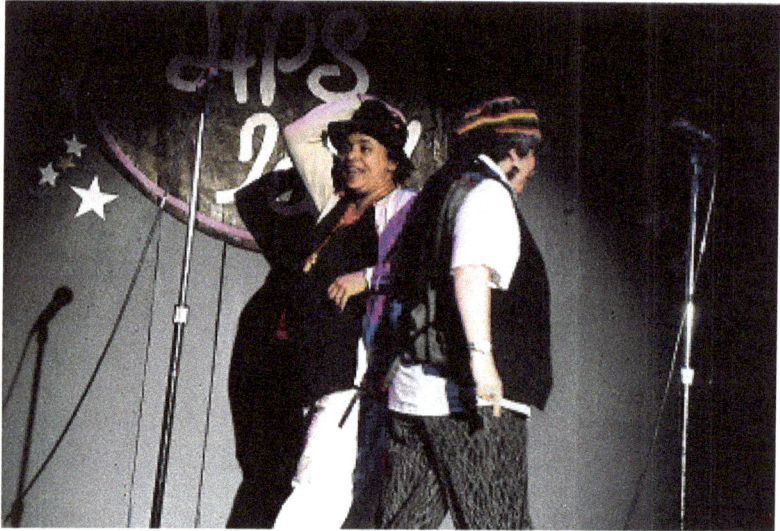

Me and Si-Si

This was a showcase for their clients and especially a showcase for my militant terminal optimism that things can get better...and they did. My understanding of Psychiatry was diminished greatly because of that Physician's outburst, thank God. God was never revocable as my sovereign Lord, and all in the wake of one Physician's exasperating eruption, I was emancipated from my mental shackles. It was my insistence, my insistence in being deep. Deep...and too smart to compromise, I took a biochemical about-face and denied every single errant thought. If it did not contribute to my recovery, it was weeded out. Period. Cognitive reconstruction. Reverse psychiatry.

Like the resident Doctor who was working the night shift at a worrier's telephone lifeline, and I, having a plethora of problems, decided to call and dump. Well, this doc was overworked. So as I launched into my most recent slant on malcontent, he fell asleep. I politely listened to his snoring for ten minutes and decided that life was beautiful. I never was suicidal again.

Logic surfaced on my ocean-face of life-challenges and buoyed on towards the now not too distant horizon.

And every time somebody asked me as to the needlessness for God anymore, I would call to mind the simple fact that I still heard voices, some days without respite. So what was different for me? I had simply learned to ignore incessant voices as though they were merely a form of tinnitus set to commentary. I lived in two worlds simultaneously, one fascinatingly wrong and the other elusively correct. And unappealingly boring. I chose to be bored, alone, without any erroneous character enhancements or imaginations gone pathetically wrong. Like my childhood fields. Alone.

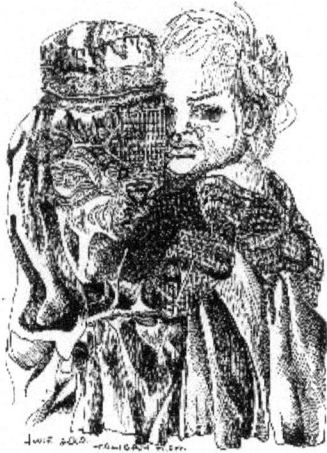

Reveal/Conceal

"Alone" was a word that I was to say in "Runaways", a play that told of teenage departures from their home life in favor of the street life...my departure was cemented for nearly forever with the word "Alone" as it meant mental illness as well as running away physically. Being so alone made me moody and impatient with people, whilst inwardly emotion overwhelmingly dictated the landscape of my surreal climate. I would dream all night about Sting and how I had missed out on revealing my psychosis-propelling vision, and

45

wake to think of him all day. He was so popular...but I sadly felt that I had made my first life blunder—while still sixteen, mind you—when I revealed that I had had a vision at all. So how long can you, should you keep a secret? I successfully developed needlessness for that rock band, and God rules. Sorry, guys...one of us got away, without breaking the "law".

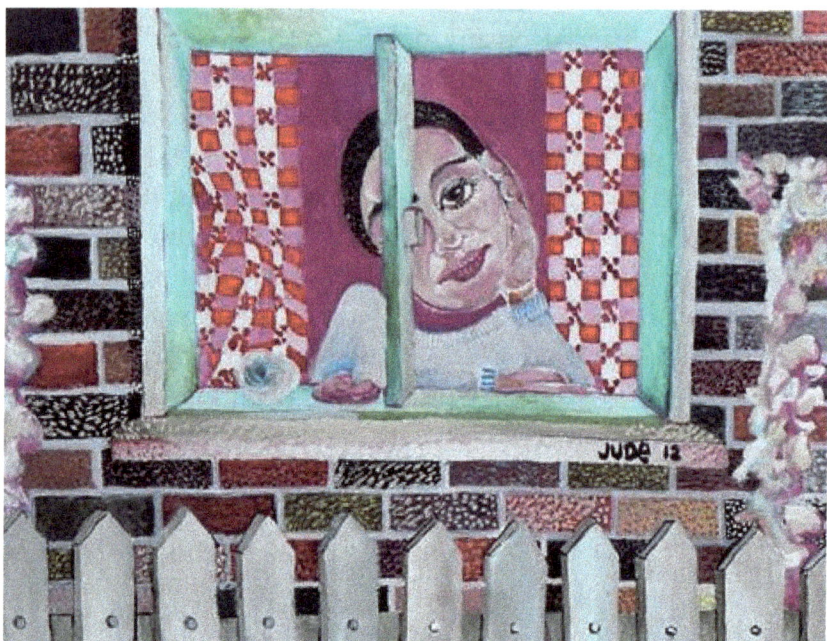

Chapter Two. Part two

"Is that my Mother on the phone?"
-Andy Summers

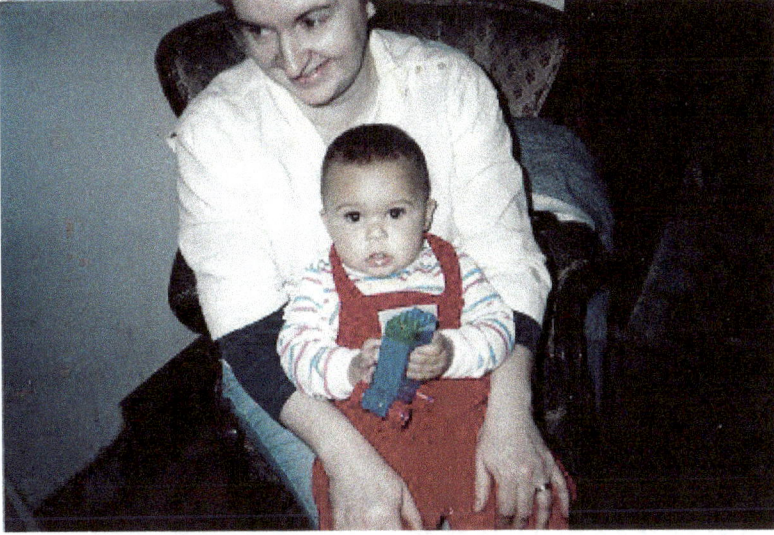

That's my Mother with Manda on a chair

So some people DO paint clouds on their own ceilings. Like John Ono Lennon, a famous rock star of the sixties. Me being a burgeoning young artiste, this kid was blessed with ample canvas and paints. Somewhere on the Toronto-bound GO bus I put on my first creativity helmet voluntarily –I had someone to protect at art college. Could it have possibly been me...? This apparatus deterred too much creative deviance (temporarily dominant) while preventing ceiling-piercing altitudes. I would get better, someday. Yet, I never did penetrate that iconic dome, alternatively spending years painting clouds galore. Loads of white clouds. Looking completely retrospectively, I do not recollect sighting ANY castles in the sky of mine. My brush, though, made the best of both sides, now and then manifesting the best fluffy, white collaboration of thought/water/cloud/genius.

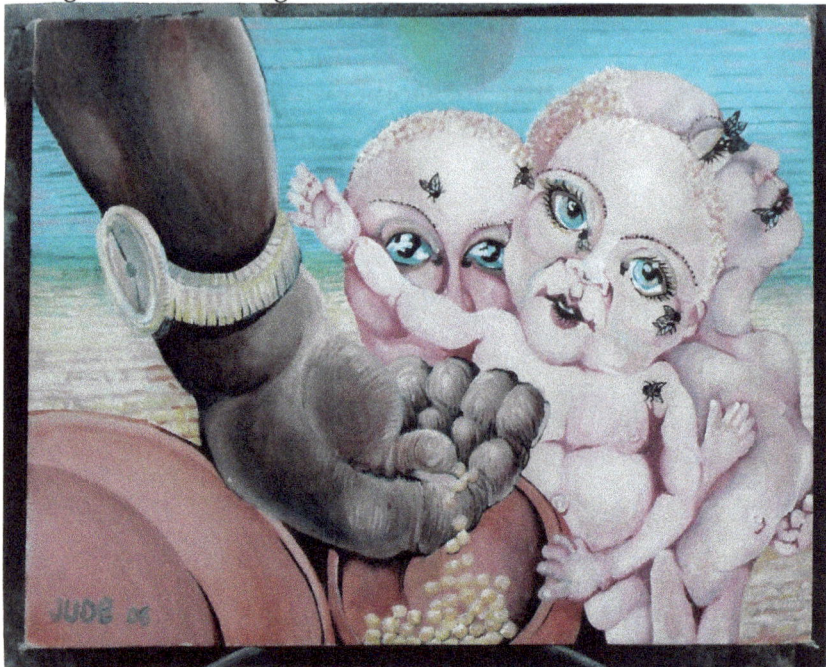

"Must be the CLOUDS in my eyes"- Sir Elton John

—as a departure for now, I was born with some kind of infection in my eyes which landed me incubated in this isolation ward for the first six days of my life. And now, many many days later, I still have residual grayish-brown amorphous shadows among the whites of my eyes. Some sort of birthmarks. I call them clouds. More effective impact that way.--

Anyway...

Normalcy is fine, but immerse I did, beneath, and into a supernova waiting to be singularly sublimate. From lowly sanity to something scary was my way. Very scary. When things inevitably catalyzed too quickly...in a Jude like manner I decided to accelerate the process of psychosis and embraced that always-full glass a tad too tightly. And that semblance of a strong structure broke. Loads of lucid thought (water) ebbed away while gaseous insanity funneled downwards from suction through my broken glass bottom. So, what happens when you have only air? Anyone? You ERR.

I was interviewed, assessed, and I must admit, admitted. It seemed to happen that fast.

My Mother did her best, and I have no real need for blaming, but by the time she got me talking to the resident Doctor, or some other condescending type, in emerge, out came a plethora of thoughtful consomme soup. It was obvious an oxomoron I'd become. Ha! It actually appeared, and I deceive you not, that Mom was the crazy one...and I prepared my mental notes with vengeful glee so I could dictate successfully what entirely was her problem. Meanwhile we waited for our audience with Dr. Diagnosis. And as I pondered Mom's looming hospitalization, I single-handedly deduced that I myself could spotlight my own covert prowess, nonetheless, seeing that my meager mind was such an outstanding specimen. Well.

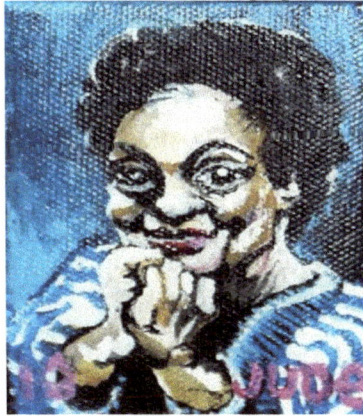

So, I betrayed immediately exactly what nature of illness I suffered from in record time: Like four minutes.

1. There were the five Careless Cast-an-idea books, read during the bulk of seven days (I slowed down for that weekend.)

2. The portable Junk, which was glossed through during the previous summer as some enlightened light reading.
3. How I was first offered, and then fed, such street drugs as would promptly render me without defense for far too many hours.

Finally, upon assenting that I heard voices, the man pulled Paranoid Schizophrenia out of his hat. At least in my encounters, I had no police record. I had burned them in a stinky rubbery mass in an old pressure cooker belonging to my Mom, and, halfway through my ritual, realized that the whole thing could explode. So the house smelled of burned plastic Police records, since I had to open the pressure cooker lid in lieu of detonating everything. Define that.

The day was March 28th, 1985. The day of reckoning.

This date was preserved due to, as I remember, interim plans of remaining at home until the emergence of an available bed in hospital. So, my bewildered one-step-previous-generation-ancestors picked up my prescription and dutifully doled out said pills. Except for one. Sitting on my sofa...amazingly feeling better so soon, I thought, entertained, and then ventured out for a safe stroll through the thoroughfares in the nearest proximity to our house. So peaceful. All was bliss until this curious muscle distress in my neck manifested itself involuntarily. It felt like someone had placed a python around my neck and things were getting tense.

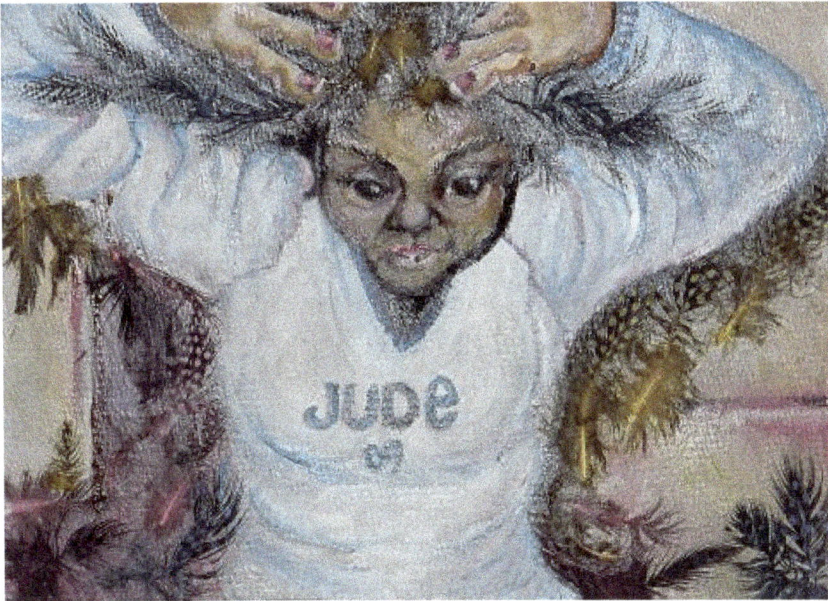

Blackbird

Terrifying head-circling. I could not stop the circles. To cry out for help with my "Tardive Dyskinesia", an overlooked side-effect created by my medication minus that one neglected crucial pill, proved fruitless. There, over there, were some people actively standing still and ignoring me purposely...there were no tablets or cellphones for years and years yet. Those erect standers at the nearby bus stop were unmoved. So I continued my homeward aerobic warm up-style walking and inevitably reached home at last. Humiliated...I could have died of embarrassment or even maybe over-exertion.(?) I swallowed my pride and my tiny little pill prescribed for side-effects which stopped my spherical around-the-shoulder experience. Lesson learned. When you are experiencing your first breakdown, always tote a hula-hoop... just in case.

Everybody at the bus stop went on to their skinny-money jobs...you can bank on it. So after much relief, I deduced to declare defeat and resume the sofa sitting with newfound motionlessness. I sat. I sat. I sat some more.

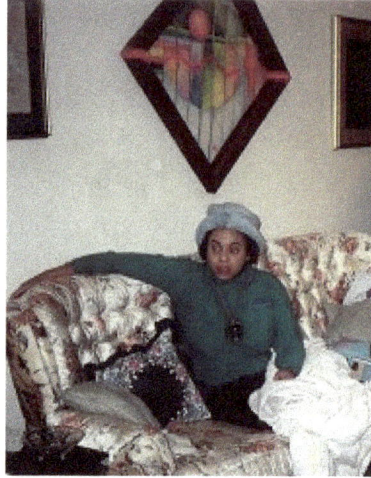

The next day arrived, redemption at last. I was admitted, yeah. I spent a conservative estimate of over one day, then a half one, side-stepping in avoidance of maybe twenty very sick and uncontrollable mental patients on some kind of hospital ward...or it could have truly been a UFO. Some were saying they were in Heaven, others in some time warp. It was hard to determine. How could I avoid these crazies that were at every turn, and smoking like fiends, and drinking cup after cup of the weakest coffee on the planet...perhaps from Trinidad Low Valley. Then I glanced, hapless, at the large, great big huge sign above the nurses' station which blabbed wantonly...

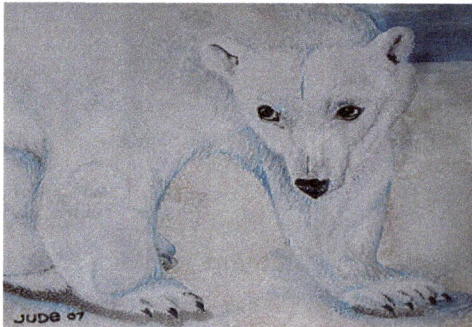

"FOURTH FLOOR PSYCHIATRY"

That, my friends, was the rub. But was it completely needed, I mean, in order to rub it in? The single most crucial puzzle-piece was "jello" nailed in by a feather like a square peg into a black hole. Standing here in my psych-cocoon, I could finally feel safe. I was CRAZY! That's all.

YAY.

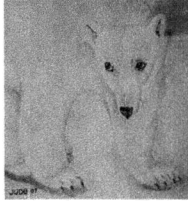

Disabled Me

So as I surveyed a hallway of this psych ward containing, like, a movie set-like payphone, on the wall, I soon detected a black haired bloke reporting the crime in progress of habitual mass poisoning by the devious psych nurses--to the 911 people at the other end of that phone cord. He was serious. I wonder if that's an actual Doctor's report, serious? Studious, I pondered my own nemesis. Not much time left. It's a good thing that time kept stopping. Doomsday loomed at the medication station (kiosk?). Then the unavoidable happened. They called us to consciousness and to the pill dispenser cart. What could I do? Quickly, I adopted the practice of planting with swift skill those prescribed poison- pills under my tongue until disintegration. Ha! The bitter acidic nature of what that guy timely claimed as a poison pill—provided the prompt removal of any lingual frenulum under my tongue, in fact. But victoriously, that horrible poison was not swallowed, and hence I was truly paranoid...so now I would only just swallow my tongue to death instead.

The next reluctant "PILL-GRIM-age" to the nurses' trolley spawned a flurry of bravery and I curtly requested the plain truth inquisitively demanding, "Is this Poison?" For the life of me, I do not recall if I received any response. Some moments are lost in antiquity, I imagine. Having no residual muck under my tongue, I resorted to compliance with my meds. Alors, I was too late.

There were more telling hurdles to encounter in my race to figure out what "psych" really meant, not to heighten the hype. Apparently if those workers-of-the-ward assume that you are not haplessly receiving recovery remedies with exceeding mirth you were named non-compliant and took a swift hypodermic needle consisting of Haldol in the buttock of YOUR own choice! I had already received upon recruitment to this army of mental deviants, a standard-issue needle.

That night I needed help getting into my flannel pajamas.

--Outfitting the unfit--

The next morning's breakfast sat untouched.

I do not think I prayed, but it was a Catholic Hospital, of course. Thank God for that sentinel with crow- black hair who timely tipped off the police. They would be here any week, now. I decided to wait and watch.

I patiently spent the bulk of my first hospitalization of six long months waiting for the police. My new occupation. (It's hard to protect an entire space-ship teeming with helpless mental prisoners-of-war, even when you have within your arsenal somebody confused enough to get the number 911 right). How do YOU remember 911?

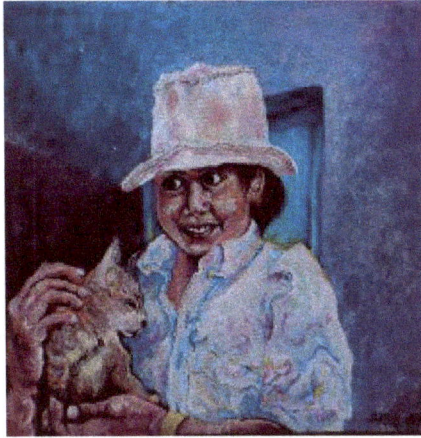

One Week Before 911

So I started noticing that people were watching me. And not through the television set. Angrily. Ever since I gave my autograph for that Psychiatrist on the bottom of his paper of printed words. (I guess he had no blank pages to offer.) He kindly provided an 'X' for me with a beautiful straight line following it, for my concentration, to write my name out. My signature, my official claim to fame, admittance of my gargantuan greatness. (So I guess I gave my consent.) And so, they studied me.

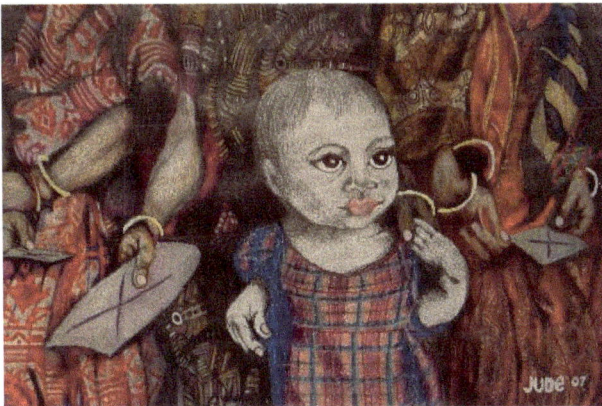

Be careful what you are signing

After that, the next important revelation was the fact that prune juice was advantageous for regularity, in fact a duodenal delicacy, to be subtle...yet the hemorrhoids manifested a painful end.

But I had lots of activities to keep me busy. Smoking. Sitting. Entering a washroom with a lighter to see if I "still" looked like Sting, with the right lighting. How original. Depositing my saliva by hand on the top of every door frame...reliving something in the Bible about Passover, or something. I would get up in the night to smoke a few cigarettes. The medication gradually would lull sleep into my life with each successive day's night.

There was this crafts room for the resident patients, where my deviant and evil (or so I surmised) art skills produced pink and gray kittens. Very scary. I guess it's hard to mimic demon possession while sojourning in a hospital run by Roman-Catholics. I made a portrait of Dr. Martin Luther King Jr. for my brother, Stuart. And of course, I spent many minutes mesmerized by a poster of a strawberry on the door to this artistic workshop. It was at least four-dimensional, popping from the poster in a super-red mutation.

Better get back to sitting.

So, there was this concert that took place with a world-wide audience that experienced it, globally. I was one. It went on for several hours, with all the best artists singing away in order to raise awareness and money for starving Ethiopians' empty stomachs and gastric urgency. I mourned my former lucidity although this loss prompted overwhelming emotion, and so I would weep while watching as well. That was the Live-Aid concert. Attended by everyone but me. I was unknown...anonymous for the entire hospitalization, and that day, also. Rub it in, rub it in. How does it feel? You don't want to guess.

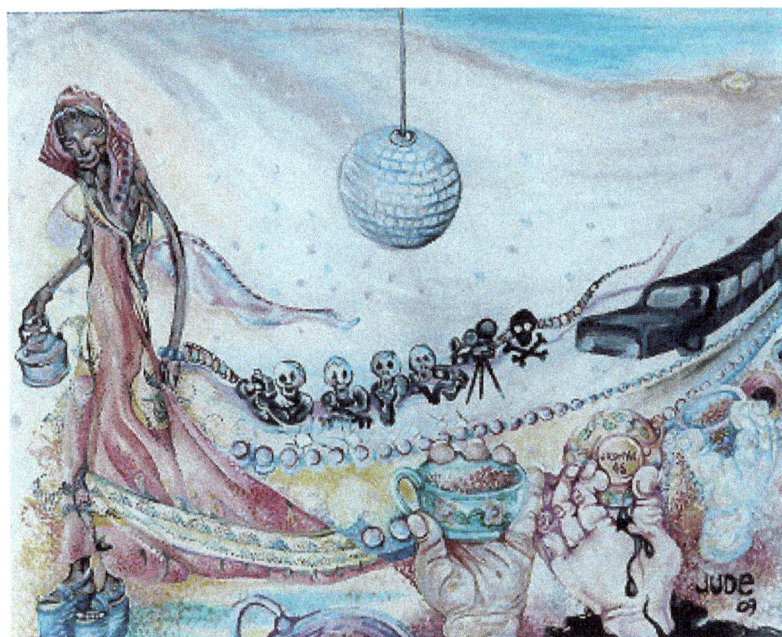

Resident-model-starving-person

This finishes chapter two, the second.

Chapter Three

"I did not shoot the Deputy"…
                                        -Bob Marley

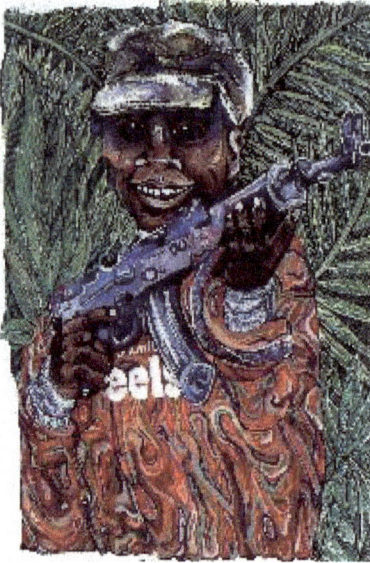

Angel of Death

Police brutality. So they have an unwarranted search decree because of your misplaced mischievous malevolent malice. And, reluctantly, it is high time to claim my own sad sneakiness. Luckily in my case, with Schizophrenia all guilt and blame are the self-same—defunct, yet ever present. After years of self cultivated confusion, delusion, illusion: all is diffusion through the cracked glass of varying levels of water. (See the illustration) Funny word, cracked. My oldest Brother always said that reality is two people's hallucinations. So what if two people cracked identically...would that constitute the existence of some simile of a doubly presenting illness?

So, folks, let's have a group flashback to nineteen-eighty. It was a tough winter for Schizophrenians, as well as fledgling crazy-types across the spectrum, just learning the dopamine ropes. John Lennon was hopelessly shot dead with five separate bullets and eerie accuracy, in the back, in an impossible attack that effectively amputated his heart from all its' attaching vessels. Evil vassal. President Ronald Reagan experienced a shooting, and came within a sliver of dropping dead after a bullet grazed his heart, missing it's mark. Mark David Chapman (shhh, maybe he will go away) and a man named Hinkley joined ranks in this threefold statistical impossibility: Two badly medicated misfits, turned to outward violence, who, normally(?), would have withdrawn into obscurity...but rather, damaged the chest cavities of two relatively treasured men, one fatally.

And, fourth, tore the heart out of society's tolerance of the mentally ill, or local screwballs, more cleverly labeled at the time. After all, they should have realistically been gradually abandoned by their buddies from High School, after graduating into nonsensical deluded inactivity. Swiftly whisked into a room in somebody else's large house. Beans 'n' franks with maple syrup for a meal. Smoking outside. Happily watching the busy money people with their skinny lives ignoring everything while they caught their respective buses. Those thin ones, disdained and negligent and resolved and irritated by the very schizophrenian presence of "us". And with every cough, it was time for us to light-up again.

Oh, and the reason for our obesity is simple: the medication makes you gain weight and so, the gradual growth of your girth is ironically a sign of recovery. Rotten diet doesn't help, additionally.

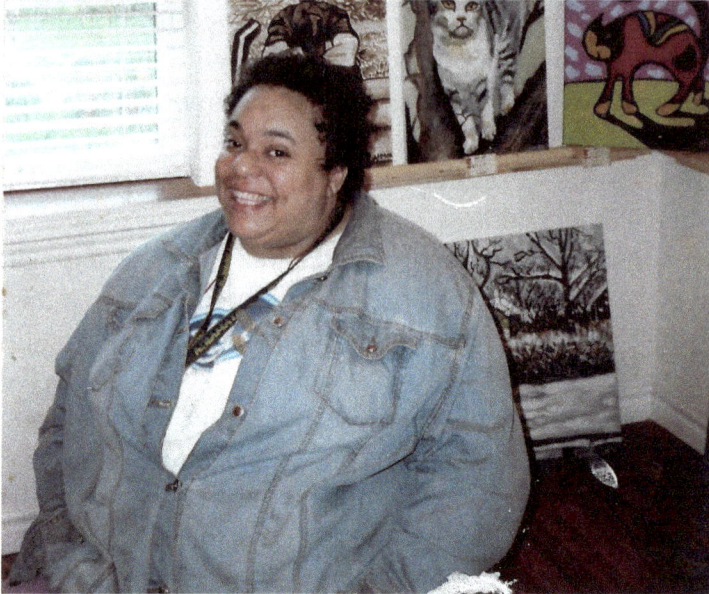

Me. Ya.

So, why did they do it? I now understand the importance of compliance and its outspoken necessity. Period. Although the rates of criminal acts among those who are mentally disabled are congruent with the percentages of "well" law breakers, bizarrity is the actual offending attribute that the public feeds off with mass rejection. We schizo's seem to do it with style, thank-you. But not today.

And so, we are compelled to cultivate boredom(which I personally love) and embrace the life mundane, as a permanent proven refuge from bizarre bursts of... stuff. House cleaning, laundry, groceries are initially our life sentence, and eventually with the advent of wisdom, our privileged pride. You see, some of us are still in lodging homes. Indefinitely.

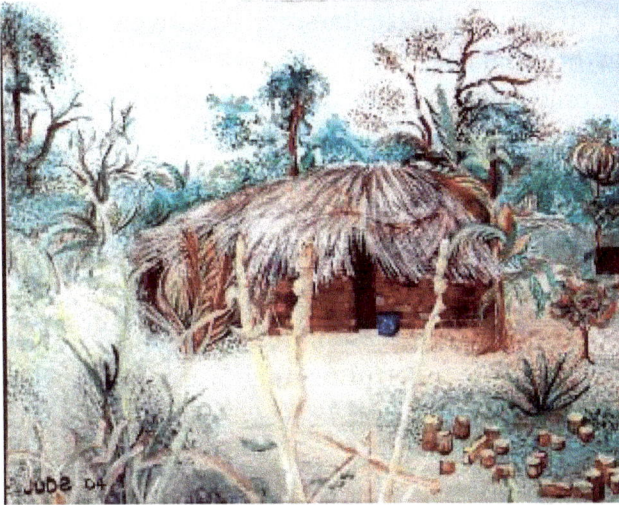

The Global Villager

Personally, I prefer the practice of humble habitation to that of "acquired greatness" and a balance of subtle minimalist home dwelling to keep things bereft of excess baggage. We two, George and I have pride of rentership, however you venture to interpret this. Sentenced to a life of marginal chores containing repetitive living skills. Beats hospitalization, any day, and wards off boarding house boredom hopefully for life.

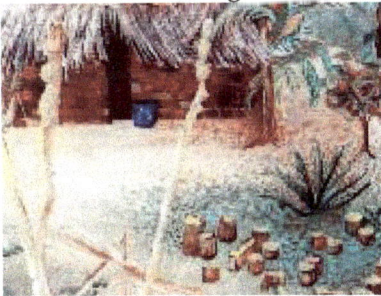

everybody hasta have one blue box

You see, hospitalizationism, a word difficult to say, is even more costly to enact for patients and society altogether. Being removed from normal social situations re-disables the progress that had been made for the dignity-stripped patient of a revolving door mentality found in society. Society, in turn, pays the price-monetarily- for an unfortunate recurrence in a psych ward. It takes approximately 900 dollars, conservatively, to force one to remain in hospital...per DAY. However the same sad patient requires only about 1100 dollars, per MONTH to conservatively live in community as an independent individual. Indefinitely. And if they are lucky enough to be prescribed Clozapine they may never relapse again...and that is an "order!" in a synaptic sense. Myself, I haven't had a hospitalization in a quarter-century. No applause, just throw ideas. When wellness swells anew like the high-tide of reason, this freshly healthy one has the happy occasion of wonderful waning of frenetic fancies. Upon recognition of restored normalcy, one is no more delusional...we don't need it anymore. At one point, "I'm sitting here in my right mind" was my preferred exclamation. Me and my Mothers would be playing Catan and I would detect my wellness reborn. To work towards being a newly revived cognitive giant can now be possible. One is no more restricted to remain seated, stubborn and sadly erroneous, but is able to adopt repetitive factory work, or hamburger flipping, or seamstress work (although it seems stressful), or housekeeping, or lawn mowing for a senior relative. Or tedious explanation of how to get someone better.

It gets better. The new generation is blessed with early high risk intervention. So, before the "damage is done" and somebody (not me, though) loses their synaptic "spark", one is granted to escape that dreaded first episode. A low-dose of
medication is initiated and the youth goes on to attend university, full-time work, marriage and baby-making...something my husband and I tirelessly tried, to make perfect self-actualization actually a possibility. I have even seen with my eyes a young couple's incredibly young baby boy that they named "Jude", for some reason.

And so, you good listeners, we all remain the unsung heroes, us nuts, saving the day for the nation's coffers every day spent in the community. (900 bucks) Co-existing with those who upon revelation of our diagnosis could spiral away flailing arms like a chicken with his head recently removed, whirling out of sight. I wish they would grow up. I've frankly been awaiting this maturation event in my own life experience...with untold silence.

So why suffer silently? Sometimes someone straddles themselves across the chasm of craziness, to only discover that it is a fine line, after all the pain, that separates us from them. They have the irrational fear of cracking up, and we rationally neglect to break the ice, cracking it being a sub-atomic no-no. They're just not ready. Sometimes the mental maze computes a solution, booting up a wellness website, so to speak. Sometimes the dam bursts, spilling out mega-gallons of answers, galore even. Sometimes this stuff gets written down, sometimes painted, sometimes sung. Sometimes by me. We all HAVE heard of sublimation, consequently, if this novel novel is to be digested, if this "concept" is to be applied onto the weeds of thought overindulgence, starving them out, then in time a bumper crop of wellness can be harvested.

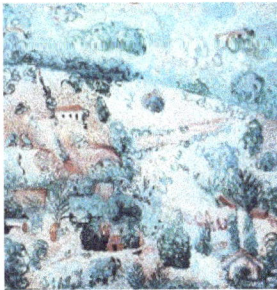

Rolling Hills

How about that tender treatise, as opposed to shooting you down, Sheriff John Brown?

Chapter Four

"Beware of wolves in a reggae-riddim"

-my saying...nice, huh?

So, after anguished deliberation, for decades, now comes the crux. Do...do I maintain silent acquiescent support of this capricious culprit or do I flush his sorry act from subconsciousness' subtlety, bringing on the day? I could not stand another night of medicated "sleep". How about a light-of-day-after-dreadful-day of morose, repetitious maladjustment? Ring a bell? I think I made my choice. Guess what it is, friend? Like many anonymous victims of virtues-turned-venom, I have voluntarily subjected my psyche to significant stinging at the hands of multiple musical meddlings. Like reggae music? I used to. It seems that someone complimented my malnourished dietary practices in my teenage years... accelerating me prodigiously towards breakdown-mode: completely complemented that fact with an absolute juxtaposition of gorgeous music and garbage-goes-in, symptoms-come-back-out lyrical genius. Some semblance of structured musical solidity, good song stuff, secured the preservation of my personal intellectual capability, although the resemblance to "psychotherapy sessions gone wrong" lyrics left me hopelessly... emotional. There's just no solution for my angst, except that I am not completely alone, now, am I? So to preserve our shared predicament, I will end this chapter. Even if I said nothing, ever again, 'till I were 95, I still would have made a choice.

I hope this is legal. The Police could come after me.

Chapter Five

"Tell me about your childhood..."
--some psychoanalyst, somewhere.

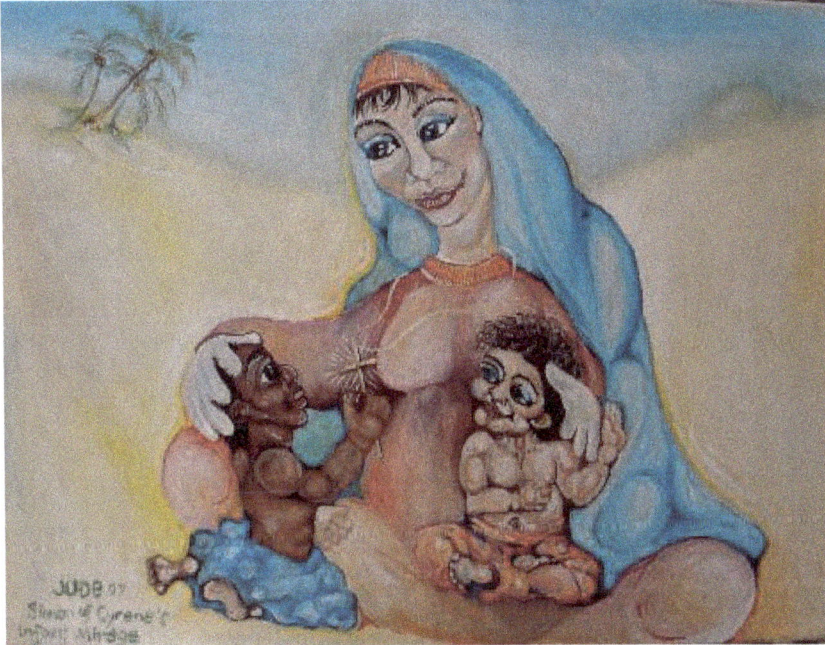

The infant mirage of Simon of Cyrene

To begin, I had nooo friends. All of my friends did not know how neglectful they were...they just thought they were playing the "Race" card for fun and were basically good people. I was the one who needed to attend Church every Sunday for years without missing, and then would receive a belting (and I mean with a belt) as a nap induction after getting home, again and again. "Stop crying, or I will give you something to cry about" was the retort falling from the mouth of my benevolent rule- enforcer known as Dad.

The inevitable introduction of that said belt would inspire me to go for my nap, where I would stay, slightly earlier than my siblings, producing a stay of execution for me-sadly for them. I only got belted three times. Clever? My siblings blame my mental illness on that formidable fact. I was too smart to smarten up. This hurt me much more than it would have hurt my Dad. (Although I can belt out a good song when provoked

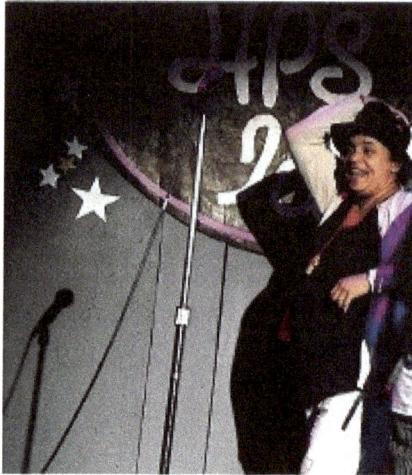

The "Belt"

properly).

So I was alone, friendless. And when I would grow tired of racial psych warfare, I would return to the fields to socialize. My best friends were of the insect-ious, wing-ed, roden-tial, ground-sliding, air-whistling variety...everything from non-venomous to vermin. We are talking garter snakes, field mice, rabbits, birds of varying levels of flight, crickets, cicadas, dragonflies, Scottish and generic thistles, and inevitably the wind, wisely wailing on its way. Everything cute or curious. My society was just and fair and cost nothing but respect for its serendipity, serving only the decidedly kind and passive ones, relenting to its beauty-full qualities. I would often retreat into the fields. God was there and He loved my lonely self with consistency. Mom would warn me not to go, but I would spend hours until my Dad's bellow would resonate through the grasses which grew all summer until they were as tall as me, "Judeh!"

So, let's talk about the fields. Allow me to illustrate verbally the essence of nestled nurture emerging adjunct to naivety...in a nice place. These fields were a refuge for one refusing to accept suggestions on how to regress into mad, stifled, racial malcontent. They say there is no escape. I had an escape. And between the waves of graceful grasses and the mutterings of winding winds, I would look up to the big sky at the white clouds: like mashed potatoes. White Cloud. That was my eventual Indigenous name, given by a Native friend, here in Hamilton, land of spewed billowing industrial waste. I have either adopted or been assigned a small group of resident allies, who have graciously coaxed something sensible out of my delusion-dotted days, and keep me connected. Had they always been beside me? Or did I summon someone from the siren-sound of my solitude? The resident Canadians, the first Canadians, and the last, of course, were those who commiserated best and most authentically with me. And remain constant, or were they always aside, my silent lamentation-sharers?

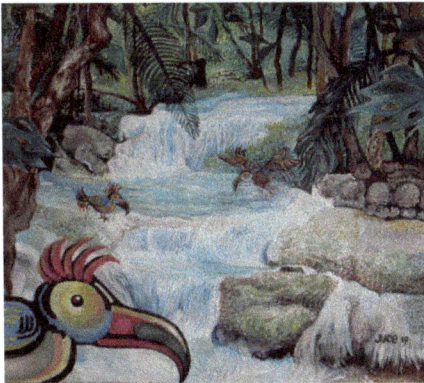

Some Sentinels

In the environs of earth and land and sky, the theater of my thoughts and everything furry, feathery, or fraught with scales and exoskeletons—these were MY fields and hapless me had hope of fielding gladly the great calling of attentive watchfulness, resilient and assenting to wherever the oblivious wind blew. No harvest of harm on my watch.

When my collective neighborhood apparently full of people collectively named "Jones" initiated a mass competition of planting in- ground pools, to keep up with other "Jones'"", their respective neighbors spontaneously produced collective wheelbarrows of back yard dirt, discreetly dumping each load into the nearest proximity of my saffron, feathery grass. What ensued was mound on mound of dirt. In an insane way they carried out a group-obsession with possessing backyard dive-in bathing holes. And so, the earth transported to my territory soon developed into rather round heaps of huddled hills that I grew to imagine were actually traditional burial grounds, and grew to learn to guard them. Since they seemed as such...I stood soldier-like, serving my Nation. I would put my one foot upon my other leg's knee-cap in a fourth-world way, mimicking my own ancestors. I don't know how I knew such things.

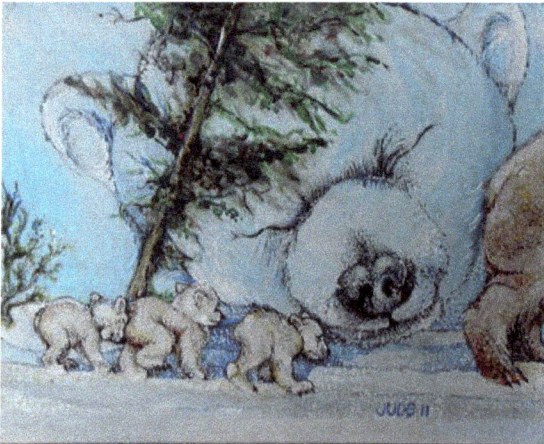

The grieving Grandmother

Speaking of dogs...cool biographical transition...there was Raquel. The most beautiful puppy on the planet, named after a famous Hollywood star, and my fave grape juice. And I treasured her as much as any ten year old could. She was opted to be the family pet, although I was the usual dog walker. Sometimes we would both visit the fields, Raquel bounding through the grass which was slightly too high for her. She was smart and learned dozens of tricks, and yet always fell for the placement of some artificial polymer poop in our rec room, left strategically where she would have the occasional accident. Upon sniffing, she realized she was proven innocent. If dogs could laugh in relief, Raquel did. Once in a while she would get away and set off down the busy Upper Sherman avenue. I would pursue in my flannel pajamas with a slippery hunk of jello to entice my pup to return.

She would always protest being bathed, as she was adopted to us with fleas present, that is, until her very first bath. It seemed that the fleas crawled up towards her head in avoidance of drowning. That freaked her out. But she always enjoyed the fluffifying hair dryer, after her bath. Warm and fun.

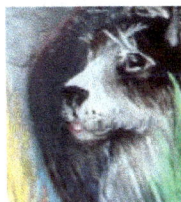

Raquel Welch Nunes

When we did eventually move to the lower level of Hamilton, Raquel was sent to a farm, from which she "ran away" on the very next day, or so the story goes. My Mom declared Raquel to be her own, ultimately. Our medium-sized mutt was acquired on the advent of Dad's bad heart condition. He kept his promise to me as well as himself, not knowing how much time remained for him, buying a nice 27" floor model COLOR television, along with the pup for me.

Dad was on couch rest, when not over working as a school-teacher wanting to be... more. So, we four kids sat and wrestled and cackled with abandon, watching that stupid coyote genius fall a thousand feet repeatedly trying to chase that ironically bird-brained road-runner (beep beep). In color. Dad would sleep and only until we children would remember to be quieter, Dad would wake up stating, "what's going on?" Why were we suddenly so silent? Dad was adorable and funny and once in a blue moon would command one of us to FIND HIS BELT. When it was my turn, I would implore, "O, Daddy, I don't WANT to find your belt!" But I would, not wanting to make him angry or something, and I would bring it to him and then sit quietly as he held his belt flat on the couch eyeing his color super fantastic magnavision television unable to rise very often to light a cigarette, even.

I was the family pusher-man who obediently cycled to the corner variety store, Sherhawk's, which was positioned roughly at the corner of Upper Sherman Avenue and Mohawk Road, celebrated formerly as the Mohawk Trail for the Mohawk nation that traversed it. I was oblivious to the obvious discomfort which Mr. Fieldy felt selling smokes to a ten-year-old, even though they were small packs, and mild, to boot. So was the custom in the 1970's as Mr. Fieldy smiled, musing shocked at the irony that a belt wielding Daddy would ask his own child to supply his addiction that could have killed him, in the presence of a color television, resting in his breezy basement couch. So, when it snowed...It was a blizzard those days.

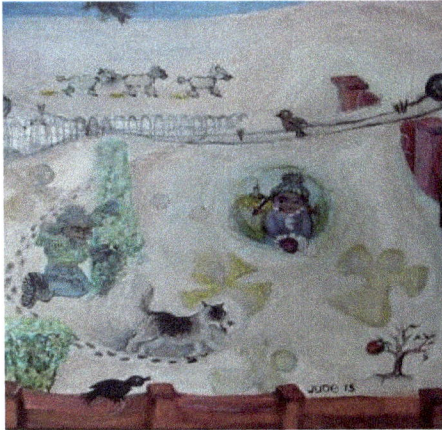

The Snow of the Year

Mom got the four of us up for an early breakfast, only to propel us outside in a poly phasic shoveling effort. You see, dad had his heart to consider, which labored too easily, and the family needed his teacher's salary to survive...so we four shouldered the clearing up of the driveway's snow accumulation, and dad shouldered the teacher's job since he was so good at...teaching, anyway. As was the custom, mom made hot chocolate with marshmallows for our well earned break from that pre-dawn group ensemble. Then, en masse, we made a return collaboration effort outside our abode. Dad subsequently showed me how to jump start his 1976 Dodge Aspen, which stalled every morn, and all winter. A nice reliable car. It was my job to place the bent clothes hanger just-so on this one part under the open hood. Every single day. So I was the hero, at least until dad drove dutiful-like to his designated classroom. Then he performed his original magic, all day long. After school hours there were about half a dozen groups and committees that he belonged to, always being hopeful for the future of the next generation.

Back to the snow.

That very snow was good for playing in, naturally. We had so much snowfall that we could dig out the drifts and make caves. What eventuated was a fear of caving caves, prompted by my mom. Speaking of play, the neighborhood kids, every single one, honed their balancing mastering on the snow-plow's displaced mounds of brown snow, and hopefully no yellow stuff. It is not really lemon-ice, you realize.

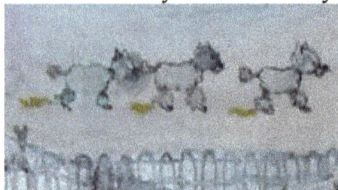

NOT Lemon Ice

Still, I did make pilgrimage to my fields, jumping over the back-fence as I joyfully responded in assent to my Mom's advice "Don't go into the fields!" --"Okay, Mummy"-- There had been a young girl, disappeared and then found in a similar field, dead, as I had been told. Staying for hours, trying to stop time, Almost successfully, if I really did try. That same time whisked me away unbeknownst, childhood whittled away, into my teenage years. But not before I met my massive mental match, mononucleosis. It started as a prompt development of fatigue, fever and a foul-mouthed odor to my family Doctor and his sniff. I was fainting in Church, having to recline in my pew. In advance of that horrific passage into adulthood, my former fields were plowed over...urban sprawl had arrived, a shopping mall and brick skinny money houses would be established, the land had been raped, I could not defend...I was flat on my living-room couch. So I slept for about two weeks straight through the Christmas holiday; you could still call it "Christmas" then. Like Father, like Daughter. I would surface to some semblance of awareness occasionally in my living room to witness the lights and tinsel of our brightly comprehending Christmas tree, and the sounds of carols on an AM radio station, only to dip back below consciousness beckoned by my combatant condition. AND, I missed every Church service that entire season. Those horrific hills and troughs-- in immaculate rows of order--- replaced my fields and upon reflection, there was no looking back. One positive realization was...the fields had become the MISSION field.

The child was grown, the dream was gone.   Right. Leftovers were fragmented figgy pudding memories and literal liberal lines of muddy...muck as a final impression of my fields.

Good thing I got out before things got any worse.

A super mall was erected, rumored to be the biggest in the world, not counting the twenty years in wait of its construction. There were other malls in the interim that were bigger, by a long shot. When the family Nunes returned to shop at the Bay or Sears, in this wonderful brick development

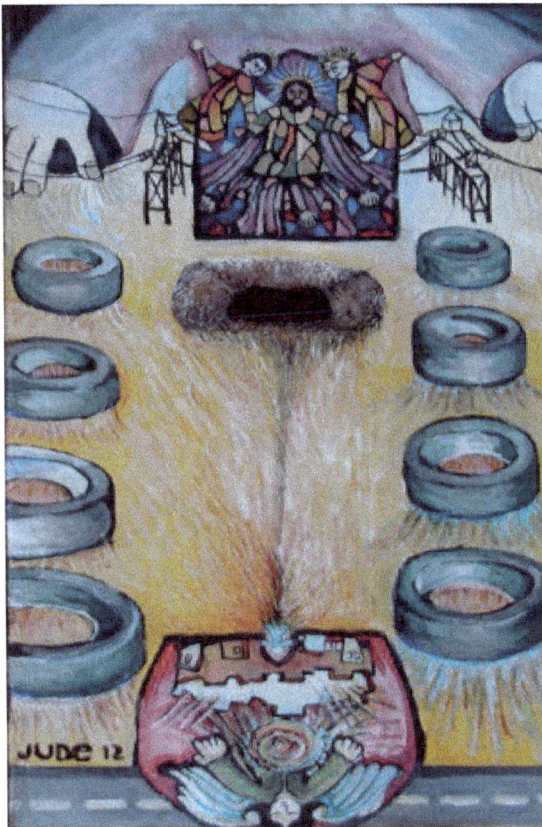

The Dream of the Mission Fields

designed for doling out our dollars, we chuckled triumphantly at a lone tree in the parking lot, intact tree-house sitting in it's limbs. So the song to sing was,

"Last Christmas I shopped at the Bay,
 I gave you a gift but you gave it away
 This year to save me from tears
 I'm gonna go shop at See-Years."

Chapter Six

"First thing we climb a tree. The Tragically Hip

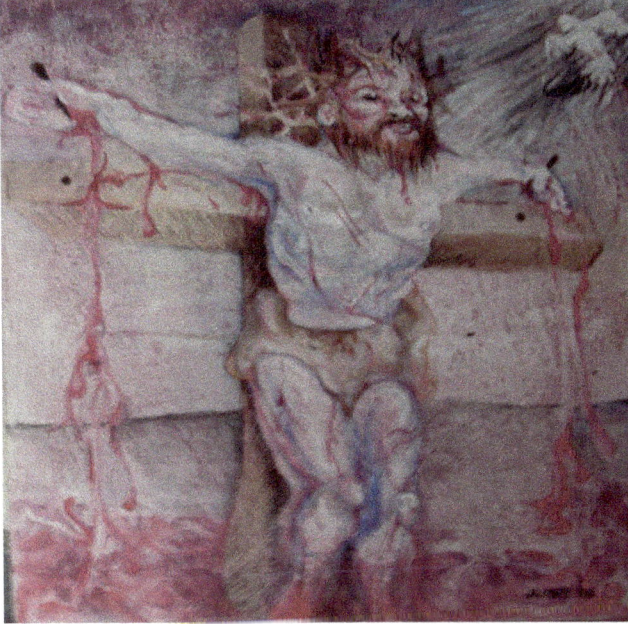

What if He changed His mind?"

The Bible says, "Cursed is anyone who hangs from a tree", somewhere in the grievous passion of our only Christ, Jesus.

So I found myself, three, or maybe four, fraught with frenzied fear as I dangled downwards from some closely grown branches, each cupping the underside of my armpits, my arms dangling dutifully down and summoning insufficient...strength to lift me even from protruding tree limbs...my little body... little effectively lifeless limbs...

...It seemed a half an hour that I hollered to whomever, "Get a saw, get a saw...", and then I saw the man in the normal fedora not even a little phased with my predicament..simply drawing near and quickly lifting me from that short tree, as it turned out... I was possibly a good foot from the ground. And this smoothly suited man was Caucasian! What? (It was post Sixties half-committed-interracial-attempt time of history.)

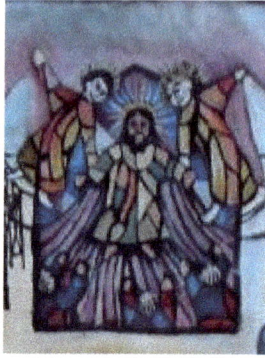

My Best Friend

Until this moment I have written little of Scott. Scott erupted into my late "sixties" life as a foul-mouthed racist four year old. On that eventful day I discovered him guarding his (all of seven trees) apple orchard standing on the land adjacent to the house his parents had rented, rightly ranting of my trespassing. As I trod his stolen land, behind our back fence, trench warfare for toddlers ceased. I called to mind a recently murdered man with "a dream" and suggested spontaneously that all should be friends. I really believed that. Still do. Harmony in the universe Maybe when Jesus comes back

All of four by that time, I had not quite surmised that all deals were off, at least temporarily since Dr. Martin Luther King Jr. had been shot dead on an April 4th morning, his legacy suffering just as lethal a blow by some generic white guy. The news footage of inner-city looting by angry, even furious people of color, held me stunned, captivated. How could people get so angry? Nonetheless I believed and maintained my stance. I had already overcome the meeting of my Jasmine Street next-door-racist-neighbour who snapped fast with a word, commenting on the nature of my brown tanned-ness.

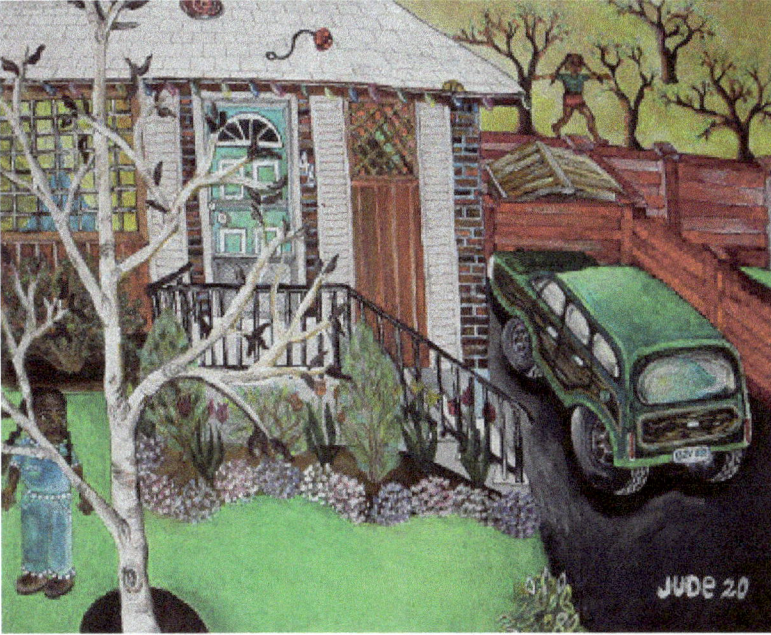

Being Brown

I simply smiled in a preschool-yet- passive perpetuation of situational diplomacy.

But Scott made short work of being won over. We succeeded upon meeting to adopt best friendship, greeting each other with close fellowship of the mutual kind. We made forts. He taught me to ride bikes, without training wheels, from the start, mind you. Hiding in the house meant for his shepherd hounds, it was much harder to exit once the two of us were inside. And the one-way door was shut. It was a nice house, insulated with styrofoam which made it even smaller than anticipated. But we emerged knowing that no-one could have heard our oxygen deprived whelps for help, anyway. That was fun.

The burnt down house was the scene of many Nuclear explosions. We narrowly avoided the fallout by cowering below

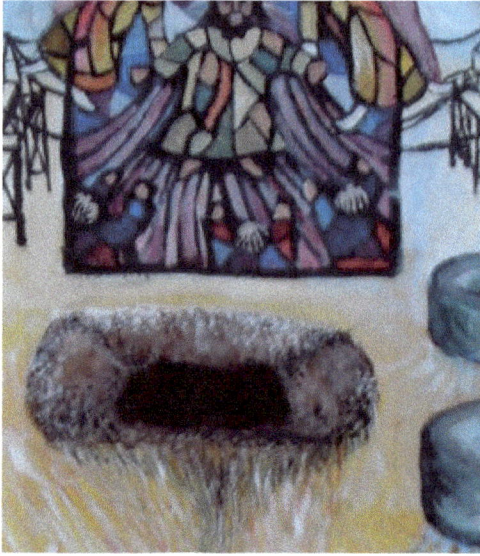

The burnt-out house-hole

Where the basement must have been. It also afforded fun for our bikes, rampantly going down and then up the crater made from many bikes, up and down the hole where there once stood a house...now just a ramp or two.

There stood, afar in the distance, a castle that we surveyed often, but Mom insisted "That is no castle there". Years later my imagination would revise, having seen that building up close, and noticing that it was a cement block factory. No more castles in the distance or on the horizon. Maybe, though, in a future sky.

And, of necessity, my first session of beer tasting, of which I had had one full sip. (my mother has never) The barn behind his house had an old rusted out mattress frame with all of the stuffing missing. It's resting-place existed precisely under the lip of the barn roof...anyway not everything affords a soft landing. Sores and deep scratches were our rewards, souvenirs to display to our tetanus-shot wielding physicians. Then there were these eerie bull horns left in my fields, yet in close proximity to Scott's little house.

They all seemed to have been removed recently from some bull and were left for the sun to initiate curing, or maybe the wind to whisper them dry. I always wondered what ritual those cows were a part of, as a section of their members were severed and cleverly placed in an anonymous sector of my fields.

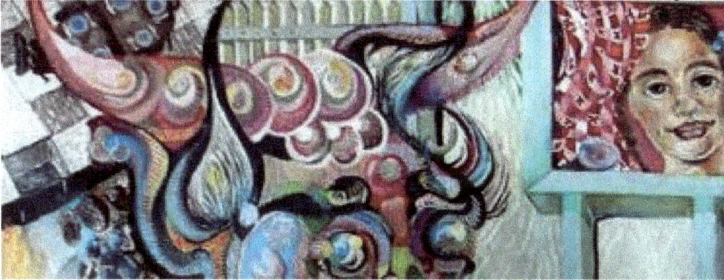

Where'd the horns hail from?"

Those apple trees in a rotting orchard plot were chosen to climb rather than reap the harvest of forgotten-to-be sprayed apples, every year bulging with more and more worms, unpalatable in their rancidity, rotten and putrid. The orchard afforded downward-spiraling inevitable inedible fruit, but fun climbing. We two best friends found once a real robin's nest cradled safely, however, little pale-blue eggs break too easily, we gleaned. Scott taught me all the wrong things, and when he left, he left little to smile about after his move out of his house, aged eight. I begged my parents to allow me to have one last session of play with Scott even though it happened to "land" on a Sunday.

What a great Little Scott.

For comprehension reasons, his name was actually Scott Little.

But I would never relinquish the little memories of a cool, poor family with three boys, an old burnt-out bus,(which they collectively had hopes of making into a road touring home), the older model refrigerator that was chained shut in just enough time to save our little lives, the occasional fort built in their barn roof infrastructure, ice rinks every winter on the cement barn floor, witnessing hawks, on occasion, jumping onto rusted metal coils from ten feet up...tomboy fun forever. Jumping over our fence to have lunch at Scott's only to be informed that it was after school had finished on that day indeed that I was to visit Scott and his babysitting mom. Sneaking into their window in order to enter that true "cellar" that had no other access, the smell of their septic tank at full capacity, the messing up of our neighbor's driveway with our bikes simply because it was not paved yet, but somehow acquired ruined gravel stones, in its gravelly stoned-ness. Sneaky circles. I truly sneaked around that end of the street for a couple of weeks, just to remain unseen and innocent until proven misc

Chapter Seven

"All God's children go to Heaven"--
Mom(emphasis God's)

So I got baptized. It's okay, I had been prepared
Theologically. Jesus STILL loves me. It is that simple. So, just as
Jesus was driven into the wilderness upon being baptized, I
ventured into my eventual story-of-life-backdrop...with my
reluctant brother, Stuart... to the fields. But wait. I, unlike Jesus
was not tempted to glory and power-without sin—I, I was
brazen and crazed about my Lord. As Stu warned me of the fast
approaching duo of definite danger, I, being consciously
baptized at four, I just knew that my newfound strength as God's
child would be enough. Stuart, wary in his wisdom, neglected to
agree with me, and was right in his fear. Faith or flight?

To the naked eye those two twelve-ish boys were just
racially rude. Until, they ventured to victimize my vulnerable
privacy whilst restraining subdued Stu. One held him back,
while the other pulled down my pants and called me names...

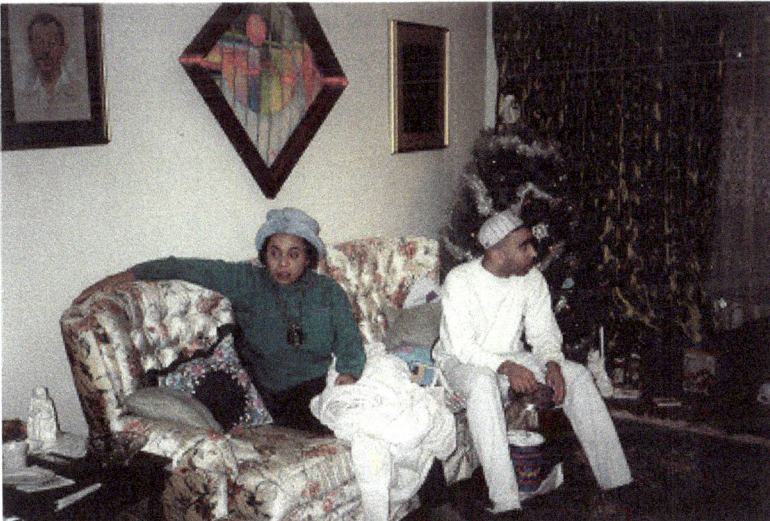

guess which ones...I screamed to Stuart to help...to help me...he could not. I yelled so loudly that I think my very soul left the scene, and then I blacked out. As we trotted back home, I kept asking Stu why he didn't help, but there was nothing to say and we knew it.

By the time we returned to our parents' house, I was convinced that that had been a rape. I imagine only Stuart recalls the tragic trepidation that took its course by those "bad boys", as they were now loathed and labeled by us Nunes'. I did not remember just how bad these boys turned out to be, but it only aided my entry into the fields most every day upon opportunity's permission, having blocked the nastiness out of

my mind and recalling the recent redemption received upon my baptized crown of a forehead instead.

So, why these fields?

The 'buzz' around the stable educated types of the time was nurture. Surrounding nature. Enveloping it. So the Home, the School and the Church remained the protective triangle that kept us young ones safe and grounded. So, it is no surprise that my respective triangle flanked—my.....fields!!!(See new illustration) AHA! I was not crazy, just safe in those forgettable fields forever remembered as I look back as creativity-inducing-childhood-enhancing grounds (for breakdown) when I had been

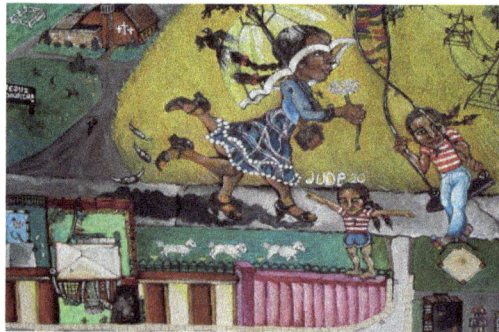

Crow's eye view

sufficiently coerced.

Home—Place of naps, and nicotine, and rice and peas, and vacuuming the red carpet of our rec-room, in the case of someone royal arriving...brother John introducing the entire neighborhood to Bob Marley's music in a morning by morning reggae concert blasting boldly in our 'burb of lower-middle-class predominately non-Jamaican suburbia. A sewing room where we laughed as Mom accidentally put five stitches through her finger, even though it hurt her. Fiberglass pink insulation that Dad and us four kids installed, and afterwards thought of using gloves for protection. The fish that Stuart let me buy on a Saturday to put in his aquariums, that would die within a couple days duration, the same kind of fish, every single time. The Christmas tree with untold re-wrapped toys that had belonged to us four before, but were needed still to refill the same gaping space under our Christmas tree with untold re-wrapped toys...Shoveling the snow- drifted driveway for our dear Dad who needed to drag himself to his teaching job to survive another day because he had had help shoveling the driveway so he could earn a salary to come home alive to rest on his back in our red-carpeted rec-room because of his heart condition...Brenna, the one who taught me forgiveness, from the force-fed "delicious" mud pies, and the little cactus which I put under her covers and laughed, to my constant verbal editorials of her climbing weight, congruent to my mocking success—Home.

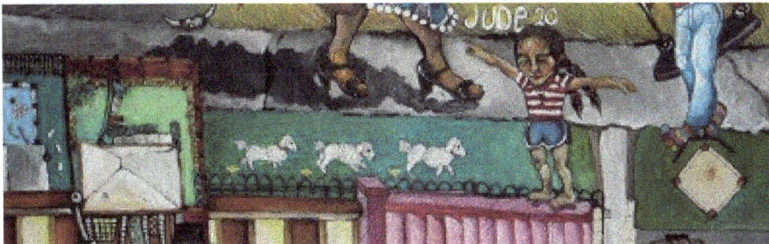

higher education

83

School—Let us go over my first day. Big brother John accompanied me down the entire block in a protective effort, mindful of my tendency to get into trouble out on my life's limb-traps in foreign fields. John walked me to the very door of the kindergarten class and advised me to wait for some "bell". That is when it happened. I was trying to seem white, stealing under the radar, but some kid caught me being biracial. He said, in Caucasian disgust, that I, in fact, needed a bath. I was dirty, I was brown. I said I had had my bath, I was clean. (This sad scene prompted future frantic soaping especially on my knees which were decidedly darker than my epidermal remainder.) Some skin, when relieved of stretching and bending, well, it adopts a concentrated pigmental elasticity darker-ness. To coin a new phrase. I knew this could eventuate into a hard day. Dainty me, I landed in the young ones' classroom(funny misnomer since the class had low class), and immediately found a sister...she was three-times darker than me so I ventured up to say "Hi" to my guaranteed new friend. She responded with a punch "Hello" to the pit of my abdomen. This CLASS was crass--School.

Church—I remember the fear of the LORD in my first attended services...The Minister would say "The LORD is in His Holy Temple, and everybody would respond en masse, "Let ALL THE EARTH keep silence before Him." Lutherans had no

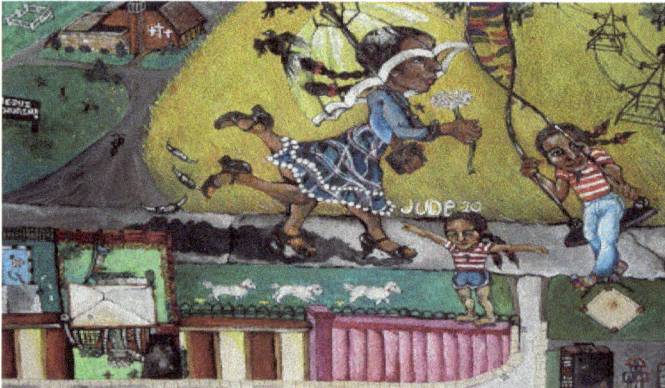

the New Illustration

problem giving the straight facts to terrified youngsters. All the earth? I better not even move a muscle. Then the reverend would say "I SAID", as though we all responded wrongly, "I will confess my sins unto God, my Father" and my Dad, the newly adopted organist would Get it "right", with "And Thou forgavest the iniquity of my sin"-sung. Wow, that was close. I resumed my extreme utter terror, knowing that my Dad had resolved that conundrum once again at this consecutive Sunday's service. Of course, after Church, we kids would tear around the building, playing hide-and-seek under the altar, in the sanctuary, to our parents' horror. Dad and Pastor had a rapport and would share with glee attributes of God's goodness for about half-an-hour after service. We kids maintained misbehavior hoping to perfect, as it were, our badness. But once in the family car, I was the one to edit our falling-short-ness as we all resumed the group argument, that would last a whole week, the starting line being the edge of our Church's driveway perimeter.--Church.

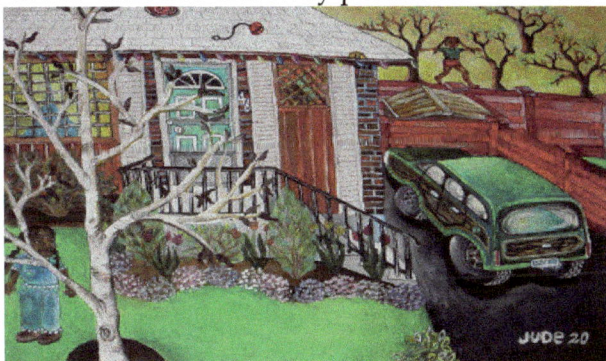

So, safe in my triangle's protection, I proceeded with my childhood. Oh, and the Police were summoned upon any need to keep any wayward child within any allotted areas. My first brush with the Police was after a game of knock-knock. This is where you knock on someone's door and then run away to watch covertly as the irate homeowners search for evidence of anyone. I was a good hider and so the mad door openers had to call the Police. I watched in awe as a single cruiser crept down our street. I was safe looking out of our front room window...scared to near death. I soon summoned the crows and crickets once again, in a world that solely made sense in it's no muss no fuss simplicity.

My fields.

Chapter Eight

"Mind if I open a window?"--Boris the Animal

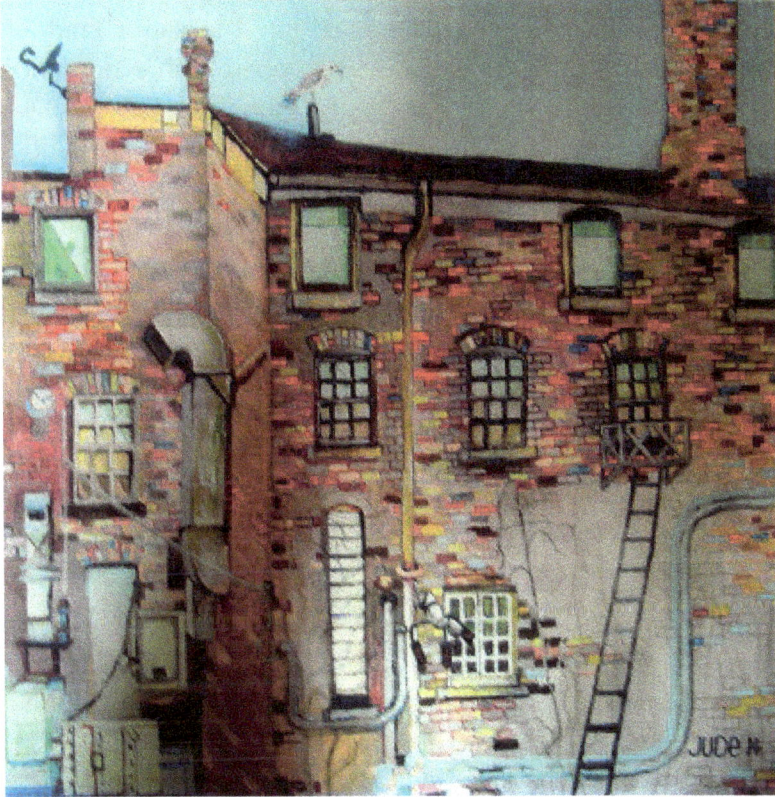

The View

So, let us abandon completely the mental agility angle and converse, reversed about my own peculiar succession of actual events re-running incessantly since their happening to this date. This, I mean, is the stuff that I knew I was wrong about perceptually, but did not care. These were various vital vignettes that messed with my blossoming youth, and decided to decompose personally, degenerating my mind into what made me...me. For instance...

On my exact precise ninth birthday my family of six, we six landed in Jamaica. On a plane. We touched down, precisely. On a West-Indian facsimile of a runway which could have sported a stop-light since it existed on the same land of a perpendicular highway-- which was stopped with every landing plane, every time, for just a minute (Jamaican time). At the tarmac when they opened the aeroplane door, there was laid out a flight (no puns flying) of stairs, leading us to crowds of stares, rare but true, people cheering. We had arrived at the main metropolis of an amazing land. When I looked to the loud crowd of rowdy Rastafarians ready to greet me on my special day, grouped on the terminal roof, I exclaimed immediately, with unabashed joy, my newly nine-year-old glee...which was met with a prompt reality-check from Mom that these cheering Caribbean citizens were, in fact, awaiting "some big-shot Rasta".

Nonetheless, the recollection of a bewildered Beatles' airport arrival in 1964 made me feel enormously special. I chose to believe me, being...ME.

Before turning nine, I was once four years old, and apparently finished painting the basement floor-red-unprovoked, which was fine, this patch of mine, even though the paint happened to be the wrong hue of red. Very funny, Mom.

So I decided to be an Artist and illustrator.

There was this one March morning, before my school careen began, when I found myself walking along the sidewalk on garbage day. Back then, there were no such things as plastic garbage bags, so we post-war fluorine-saturated-water-drinking peace-lovers put all of our waste collectively in the selfsame paper bags that the grocery cashier had provided for the purpose of carrying our specific stuff home. In the first place. So, there was a cycle of good stuff going in our house in paper bags, then being consumed, then the bad stuff going at the foot of our driveways for those collecting men, cursing at paper's inert flimsiness every time. Life was so simple and complete back

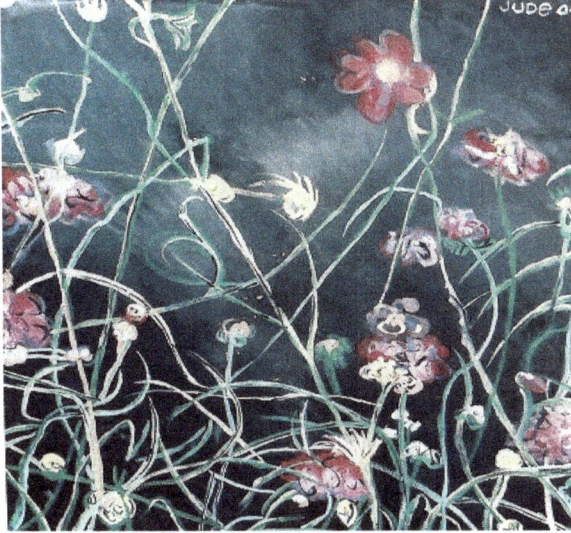

Some Art

then. Anyway, I noticed suddenly that our neighbor's specific refuse didn't stink. Enthralled, I ventured closer to discover that their personal pile had been placed in an empty laundry detergent box...hence the spring-fresh scent. I took off inside our house to announce incredulously "Hey, the garbage smells really good!". Mom had an instant comment to share...something shrill like, "Garbage doesn't smell good...garbage is disgusting...don't talk crazy! What are you, crazy?" At least I was being reared within the parameters of normalcy.

Did I tell you the one about my flying ability? Commence laughter at will. Of course I couldn't fly, except in my sleep. One Saturday evening my brother John babysat us siblings whilst Dad rehearsed the organ at our church. So there we were, four, in the basement, playing Saint-like, (since we were not in Church after all), and there was this half-wall. It ran down the center of the basement, red-painted floor now covered with bright red carpeting, red rugged cement floor... not conducive to successful flight-landings...my brother made a false move momentarily and I, musing that he was in pursuit, giggled giddy and silly-like and my feet left the half-wall in full "flight" formation. Fantastic fantasy flight. On my way down, which started immediately(?), I noticed I was in a direct collision course with Dad's expensive Lloyd's stereo system. There was no time to radio the flight tower or survey radar, and I knew what was to be done. I changed my trajectory, in mid-air, mind you, so as not to smash my Dad's expensive Lloyd's stereo system. The horrific collision was thwarted and I landed on a dime with my right elbow.

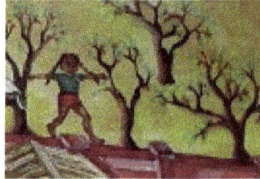

On the fence edges

It was a green stick, my fracture, and I immediately announced, with newfound magic-realism, "It's broken, It's BROKEN!!! My brother John in his Born-to-be-Minister way, made an attempt to heal, from instilled instinct. Next thing, we were all in the dining area upstairs, everyone taking turns at holding my arm up. I was so caught up in my failure to fly...I neglected to adopt support when it was my turn. My arm dangled loosely, my family's mouths gaped incredulously, and my Dad took me to emerge. (which would emerge into my life in future years), immediately.-- It's not funny! My funny bone can vouch for that.

Anyway I was in traction for three weeks, and after a couple of procedures, I went home with a pin in my arm and water in my lungs and self imposed physio for negating future flexibility fears. After that ordeal I reserved flying to being in my dreamscapes at night. I really thought I could fly.

So, Race-relations had picked up for me by grade three, not seen by me. The very same kid that said "YOU need a bath!" was asking in an offensive gesture,"Do you want some chocolate?" Well, I lost it and stamped my racist-response-temper-tantrum loudly and clearly in his ear until someone with authority came near. I reported, convinced, that "He called me Chocolate". He disagreed, but I won that fight, lost a friend, and missed out on some good chocolate. Ha! Nobody calls Me chocolate. Nobody did.

The Beatles, a lovely group of young chaps, were all the rage and therefore made people, not me, crazy. The only thing they really, really, knew about this band was that "Hey, Jude" was not written to me. I disagreed demonstratively that I was the only Judy since Miss Garland...the other one... had died. They unanimously advised that the JUDE in question existed in the form of a boy, with the name of "Julian". Yeah, right. Yet another deluded misunderstanding to defend at a later date against the flow of psych meds in my system's veins.

Did I ever hint, also, that upon reading "The Catcher In The Rye", in 1978, that I had felt a little similar to Holden Caulfield, even identifying with him, but having no logical proof of my premise, I had immediately abandoned such an obvious mental mishap.

Next came my major mental mishap.

The patterns of stubborn delusion were part of my personality from the start of my young life, something unseen until the stress of teenage angst gone awry gave everybody a good look at just what early onset Schizophrenia resembled. My young adulthood was misrepresented in an effort to follow brother John's experiential infatuation with reggae music. But by 1983, Bob Marley was long dead, John was in Lutheran Seminary in Ann Arbor and I, I was waxing and wasting mentally with no idea how to be young and biracial.

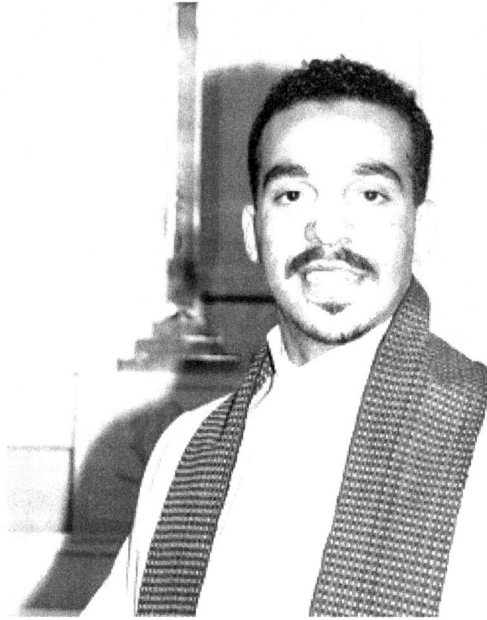

So I listened to alternative reggae, penned in (no pun needed) by Sting and the Police. This stuff was musically compelling whilst emanating, sadly for me, an incoherent subject matter-compared with the logical order of brotherhood by brother Bob and the Wailing ones.

You need to know that prostitution, suicide, underage sex, and stalking had hardly ever even entered the mind of Bob Marley as good reasons to write ditties. So I adopted a rasta stance based on what was there...some guys' attempt at worldwide psychotherapy at the ears of the ever-increasing fan base of unaware human masses. People loved this stuff, and I personally could not get enough, because it was a conundrum to me, an unsolvable labyrinth for my lucidity skills, not yet developed nor deployable. I was certain beyond a minutia of differentiation that Sting was continuing the saga of Bob Marley's shortened life. That was then. Now, I blame myself if I ever turn up the volume for "Every breath you take", because it takes me right back in an instantaneous mini-breakdown, to where I sat in Toronto, alone, on a red wooden chair for children.

"...Breakdowns, call them breakdowns, go, so, what are you going to do about it? That's what I'd like to know..."   --- Paul Simon

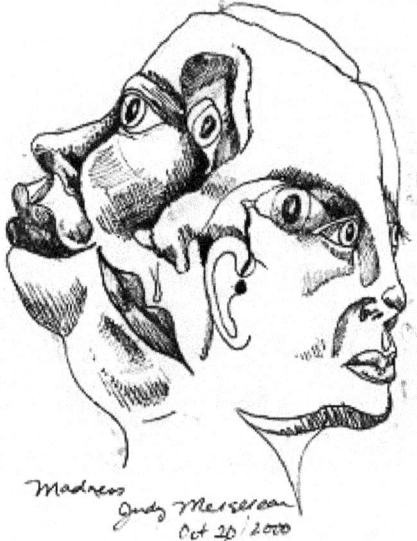

Madness Judy Merseroau
Oct 20 / 2000

Another relapse?

Another fantastic tidbit of reality remains that young women do not typically break down until they are 25 to 35 years old...I was Schizophrenic at Sixteen, hastened to my malady by diabolical genius. Now, at 53 years, I feel that I have run the race far enough to catch a "Breath" and look back at how far I have traveled on my walkabout.   I am clearly past Oshawa and turning the corner on Peterborough, and if you look up these places on a map, you are truly crazier than me.

So, six months. Paying my dues for wanting the world to have "One Love" I had sat like a louse in that lounge on the psych ward for the entire Live Aid concert, an anonymous medicated nobody.   Loads of tears for one great lost mind, disabled like an atomic love bomb. (that would be MINE to cherish) My breakdown is what really changed my life, for this was the sole mental maze I ever completely solved.

.... yay.

Weeding weeds of thought

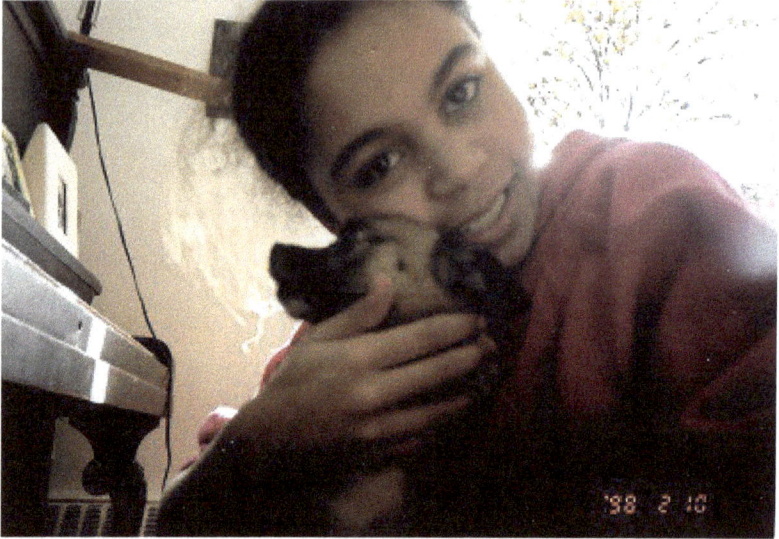

.

Skinny Pup

If you feed a skinny dog, He'll turn round and bite you, you know, so I guess that's why so many skinny money people thrive amongst us overweight lunatics who never would think of culling out your sorry butt. Even if we had a plenteous reason to do so.

Chapter Nine

"WHO KNEW?"--Pink

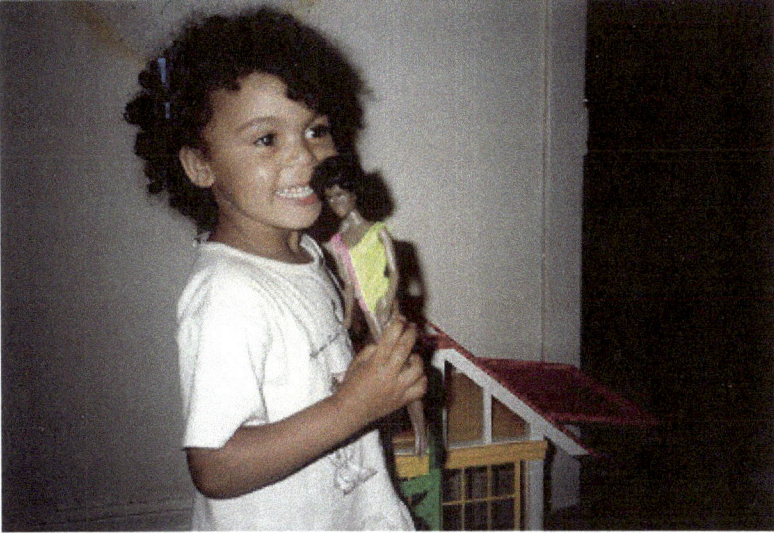

Age Appropriate Amanda

GRADE TWO. Being completely apropos, have I touched upon the fact of my childhood Genius? It morphed one morning, when it was minus forty or something similar, I cannot really remember, since the entire of the British Empire was switching to Celsius from Fahrenheit... absolute ZERO on my perception, I was spewed out of our home in a poncho down that huge long block between my home and school, thinking that I wanted to be Home schooled that cold day. It was a field day. It was a field trip day. Do not get excited from the word "field"...this was nothing special to me. My grade ONE teacher deduced observant of the lack of temperature that a poncho was not a good "fit" for that day, so as befitted a wise mind- forming-woman, she proceeded to have an actual "fit" and put me in the grade TWO class. Do you foresee what was looming later that mourn?

It was test day for Miss May's young mathematicians, and I had been swallowed into the supposition that it would not hurt to participate in such fun. It was a times-table chart that alerted the Thornbrae School primary teachers that I was smart, since I received 100%, with no mistakes, mind you. And that was grade TWO!

So they put me in Miss May's class; she might have been the Queen...I am still not quite sure. She had a grueling ritual of Pledging Allegiance to the same Queen in that picture that was hung one full foot in front of my desk. Then we would display how virtuous we had been the preceding day by tallying all the chores and practices we had achieved only to report it with a 'dot'. That dot was one of many colored in on a clown's costume, one per day that we had remembered to brush our teeth, bathe, do homework, eat our entire supper and get to bed by eight P.M. I could never remember if I had remembered all that, but the Queen was watching, and I loved to color...so many days may actually have been erroneously Dot-colored. If I ever meet Her Majesty, I may not get away with untold excess toothpaste leftover from the night before, but I might actually get

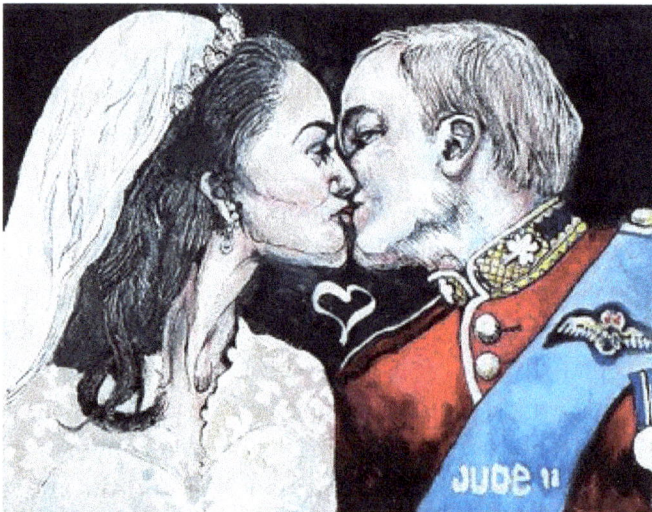

The famous Kiss

away with the whole facade... if only she notices my dotted-clown-poster first. This is my only hope.

I had been precocious since forever, my art career beginning when they noticed my insistence on being left-handed, hence possessing the creative tendency as my right-brain dictated. So my initial scholastic creation was a subtle take on potato printing. My stance was that, although we kids went to great lengths to cut a perfect print-image, life was not always so. So I ventured to twist my print in a circular fashion, that was enhanced with perfect distancing of color so that not one hue touched the same one, anywhere NEAR. My potato painting was a hit, and my Father kept it at about one foot above his desk at home, for years and years. Dotted and deliberate.

Poor Stu. Together, our sibling partnership was ne'er do well. We just could not win. As I accelerated into grade two, mom thought it best that Stuart be kept back, the same year. So if you know your math...we two were in grade two with two years of age between us. And nobody gave a number "two".

Challenge: Evolution versus Creation. Vain imaginings versus Biblical truth. The teachers at Thornbrae Public School wanted all of a sudden to understand the history of creatures,

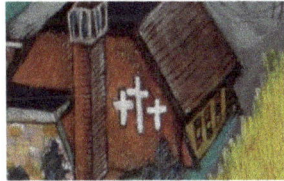

and so queried of myself, obviously artistic, to illustrate. HA! I chose the evolution of the horse, involved my best representation of every stage, and this epic mural was put in the entrance foyer of my school, to teach the children. This child knew better, however. When the faculty summoned my faculties about gradual evolving in a linear and successive sequence, I simply announced that 'the horse was created and born to the left and grew up to be on the far right. An adult equine' HA!(a Jamaican word of victory, usually accompanied with a thump on the kitchen table). I guess I'd proven Creationism. For good.

Then it happened.

That little girl that was so pretty, and pinned her penned poetry on the display board at the back of the schoolroom so sweetly, she inspired an initiation of cuteness copying. So I reached up to the board and went on my tiptoes and being one full year younger than all of my class, relieved my juvenile bladder. I had asked the teacher to be excused to visit the washroom, but was turned down as Miss May cited self control to be lacking. Maybe next year, but not as a six year old among those aged seven, Your Majesty(?). But what a relief.

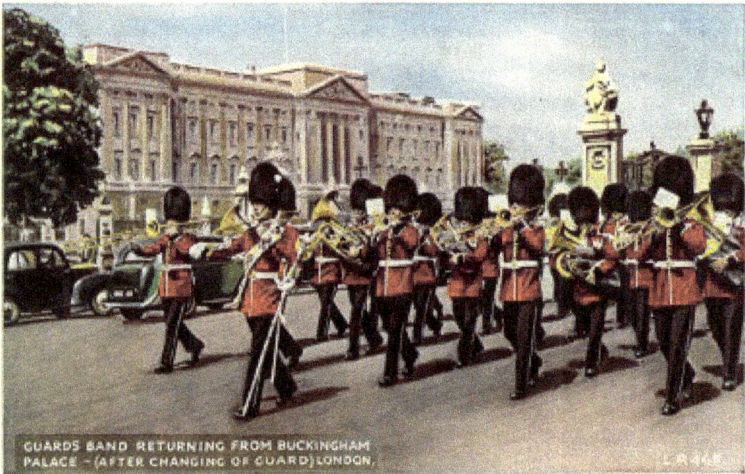

GUARDS BAND RETURNING FROM BUCKINGHAM PALACE – (AFTER CHANGING OF GUARD) LONDON.

So I marched single-file to the teacher's desk at the front of the class and curtly reported something like,"Those school mice have had a group pee at the back of the room again". She followed, and concluded condescendingly, "No MOUSE did THIS." Well, I really had to go badly. She asked me coldly "What happened here?" I, forever clever, responded,"Would you be angry if I told you?" She chillingly dictated a cleanup detail for my little humiliated hands.

After cleaning up my own pee, I returned to my desk,

front-row-center to the Queen. GREAT. Hey, I wonder what she...does?

There goes my Order of Canada. I will say three pledges of allegiance to the Queen, and draw in a few dozen clown dots to be safe. I really need something to placate my late Father, though I am the one that is late to be great.

Chapter Ten:

DEAN

So my sizable art career emancipated me from any unneeded childhood social growth in happenstance, having no friends. No growth, just artistic genius. Socialization was personally understood, but gross loneliness haunted this brown but brilliant one. I had no friends. Dean was my primary primary-school whipping-boy-child throughout, seeing that he also exhibited superior art skills. But who was more superior? So, the games began. One year, I succeeded in a Creationist mural on Evolution- from birth to natural adulthood...the next, Dean made the cover of the school yearbook. One, I was putting stickers on a massive paper, printed to put stickers on, the next, Dean was given a set of 5000 or so "Prismacolor" pencil crayons. Merely the best in pencil crayons. Dean also had a Robert Bateman print proudly placed on his parent's living room wall. Well. Well, I successfully won the winning crayoned bumblebee

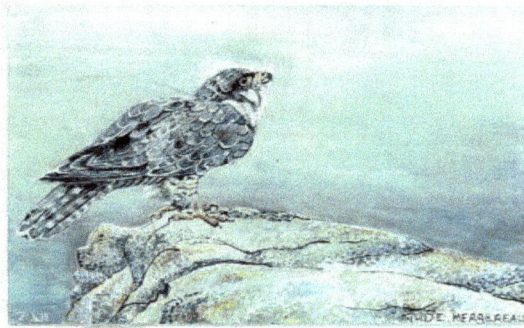

Fake Bateman

for the school newspaper...edited by my brother John.

We both had Saturday morning Art classes at the Art Gallery of Hamilton, a cultural fixture in the downtown core.

Funding ran out...we were kicked out to create for ourselves. Next step, High School. We both attended an excellent secondary school for heightened creativity, together—neck and neck to the end. Dean, as any NORMAL teen, discovered street drugs and missed countless minutes of classes, smoking cigarettes. He prodigiously predicted the decline of Disco music, and to my horror offered me an example of the new wave of music of a band called "U2". Music about war and bloodied Sundays. Get real. I, however, peppered my curriculum with outbursts of lonely crying, careful avoidance of conversation lest it lead to gossip, and mailing Bibles to my one-sided love interests. These students did not endear the appeal of my zeal. Three strikes, Jude's out.

Dean had become brother Stuart's good friend, and mine also, though in a critically artistic kind of way. When the time came for us to consider dating, I backed out, stipulating that I would only want a virgin. A virgin guy. Hard to find.

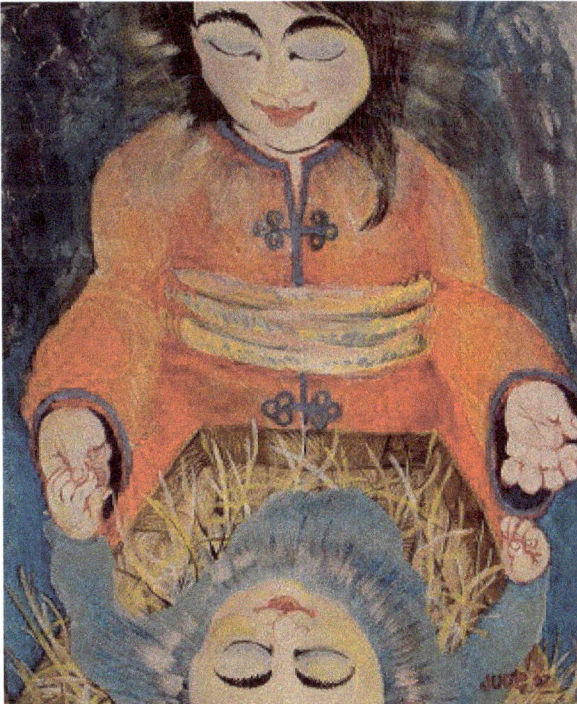

In the end, I graduated with a slightly better grade than Dean, and so received the most awards at commencement night. Honors, Proficiency, Art award, and of course a High School certificate with about seven extra credits. My parents, who had had an argument that eventful eve, remembered a camera, but forgot about film. PERFECT. Humiliation for four times at the front of the stage. Few took any snaps. I certainly snapped at the chance to scold my parents, though.

Anyway, I proceeded to have my first of five or six breakdowns...and Dean became a professor at the oldest University in Hamilton. He might as well be the Dean of English. I failed my single one course in McMaster—Religion. Go figure.

"There is one mystery, yeah, I just can't express...how you must always give your more...to receive your less...
...like one of my good friends said, in a reggae rhythm...don't jump in the water...if you can't swim... well I want you to straighten out my tomorrow."

--Bob

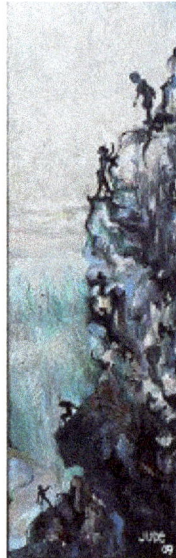

Abbr. Into. Alrgt?

Before this second book begins, I'll have everyone know how successful the jotting of book one was for me. When I began I was predominantly angry, frustrated and despondent with the life of prodigious genius gone by the side of the road...so I imagine that I hitch-hiked aboard one sane thought vehicle to another in a hippy-like succession towards better living. And as to why so much of a deluge of unasked-for emotional angst lead me in record time to nothingness, I have no answer to this day. But first I had to start somewhere...

Book Two

Chapter One: How I Met My Mother

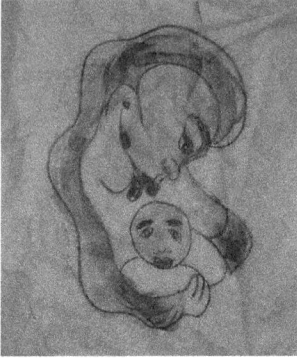

My Mother, My Baby

So, T.O.

Picture me in art college. When I could remember that that was why I was living in a city with more than 2 and one half million strangers. For posterity's sake, I was still surveying my fields.

Toronto is a cold city. As a venture in misadventure, I set out one morn to perform my personal "Walkabout." That is an Australian Aboriginal term, I think, coined somewhere, sometime, in a book I once read and took to heart. It was a room in a house that I embarked from that day, the day after a landslide federal election which granted someone named Mulroney Canada's top job. I stood stunned staring at the news in one of those red newspaper strong-boxes, apparently protecting the facts inside it, appalled that I had neglected to vote. My wanderings, initially purposed for the pursuit of this generic rock star, popular at the time, named Sting, suddenly had a mandate change, and I decided there were more important fish to roast. Stinking greedfish.

Toronto was freezing in November and I wondered, "Why don't they heat this place"

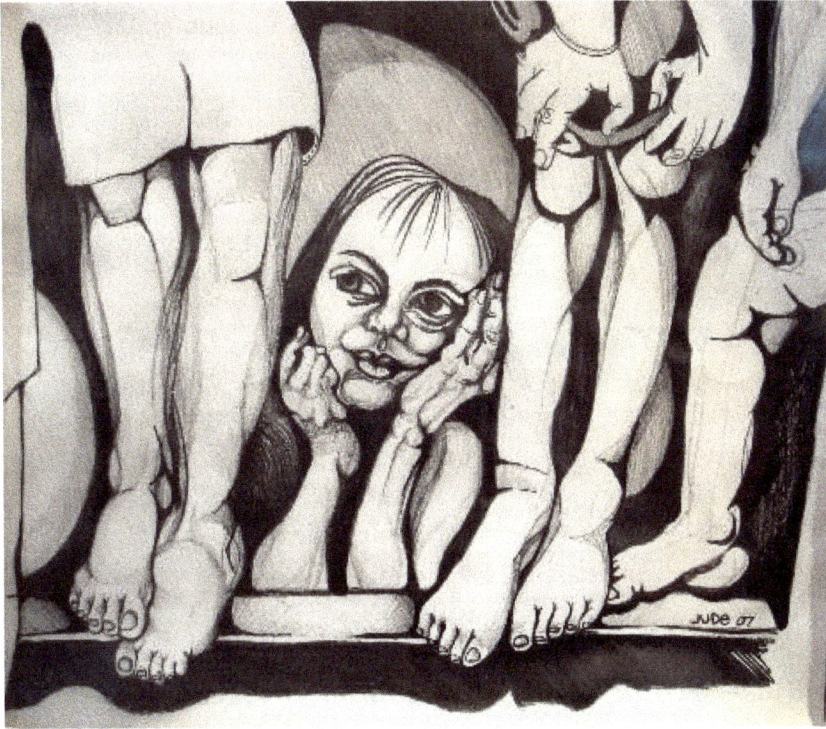

Incognito Cold

So, I slipped into a variety store, all of two or three blocks into my trek. In the room's middle there was a little child's painted (red) wooden chair, about which I queried, "Can I sit?" The young Asian girl assented. Must have been about the same age, eighteen years. Living in this Land, Glorious and Free, Kept by God. My GOD, so far being free was not so glorious. The core of my being was frozen solid as I, stolid, began my slow shivering thaw. That comfortable one prompted a decisive exit by chirping coldly, "It's not that bad". How rude an announcement. I left. At this point I would become so relentlessly cold that that memory haunts me to the present day...to the bones. Don't venture into winter with just a jacket and a fleeting dream-idea-quest in tow.

The reason for my being so very cold was simple. I wore nearly rags. Forsaken, with sockless runners that did not fit and cut into my heel, I adapted my gait to these maimed feet of mine.

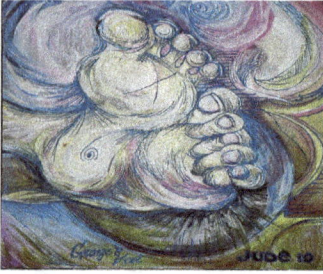

I also had very few belongings, left in my room, (which was immediately chosen upon viewing it, the first one shown.) It had a skeleton key for the door; there was no method of locking it from the inside, so I was definitely defenseless. Although my possessions were safe all day while I was away at art college. There also was an old-fashioned radiator which had been painted many times over and therefore only warmed my room slightly since the turning-thing was stuck. A red light bulb was screwed into the only source of...light, that was cleverly mounted sideways just above that rad. The window had a crack on a grand scale, and there was a twin mattress on the floor. A wardrobe closet held my few duds and an arsenal of cornflakes, my staple food for then. No need for a television, a phone...they were not worth the trouble—a funny word, trouble. Usually, when you are IN it, there was a precious something that was not worth the trouble.

Anyway, all this mess meant that my Mother, beleaguered, had no way to reach this art brat whatsoever for whatever reason.

Toronto lasted for approximately two months, and then two more weeks until the creative clever "me" ran out of bright ideas.

1. Rent the first room you view, deciding on the content of your "miraculous vision" experienced instantaneously.

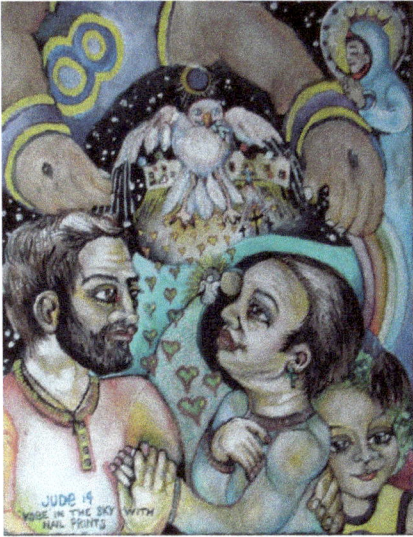

Dreams of Catholicism

2. Ignore the geography of your new nest, a hefty and healthy hour and ¼ walk to art college.

3. Refuse to use rapid transit.

4. Having no phone, rely on telepathy to contact family members on the same evolved frequency, if personally possible by them, naturally done by you.

5. Give all of your parents' money away, especially to drug dealers who dabble in recruiting young things for exploitation.

6. This should be first among rules: never apply for government assistance, ever. Let Mom and Dad fit the bill. No college loans asked for...previous generation family members punished through the nose.

To abridge the reason for my roaming travels, I assessed the spartan happenings thus far: I left. I read. I got cold. I sat. I left again. So far a momentous morning. This alternate reality business was captivating—Carlos Castaneda was apparently right! Those perceptive paperbacks he had penned-out had given a giant head start to Jude's great initiation into the Fourth World—that of the Indigenous ones, planet-wide. However, I remained in the (alternate?) reality of the municipal principality of the city of Toronto...that was my backdrop of choice mistakes.

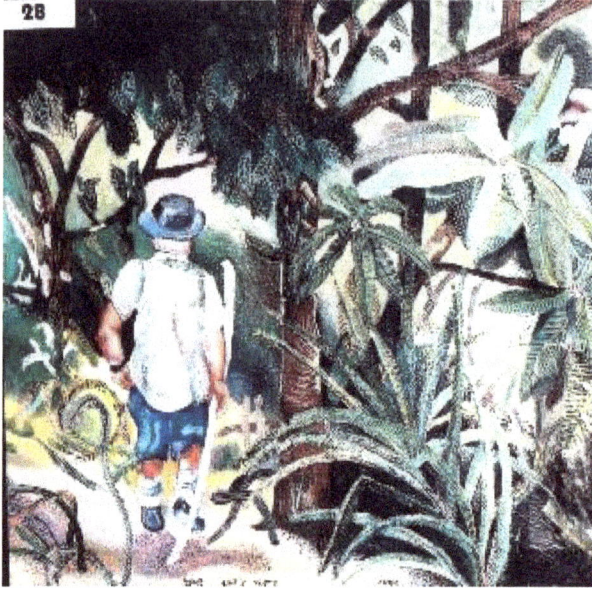

...It's a Jungle in there

There was something, I mused, of birds in their flight, ushering me to that special destination which ordinary people had no clue of existence...it was as if I were in my fields once more, but this time I was also in a huge, strange town that was brimming with spurned mental types. Toronto was cold. So I followed the birds as they moved unified in flight across this street, then adjusting their course, as unpredictable as me, to traverse that other street's expanse, and I had arrived in Castaneda-land...a place of fantastic wonders. Yes, my brain was also saturated with whatever those guys would feed mindless-me in the form of drugs.-they were not of the prescribed echelon.

Then suddenly there were the clueless wonders walking

to work...the skinny-money-people headstrong and approaching me. I did what any honorable street person would do...I crossed their path purposely cutting off their particular plummet to perdition, maybe saving their souls, or at least slowing their slide into Sheol. They did not miss a single step, even seeming slyly conditioned to droves of dream walkers. Otherwise known as persons with no fixed address. Disappointed with my ignored demonstration of denting the destination of dummies, I determined to stay the course, anyway. Not even fighting corruption on an individual level, one nail hard money-nut at a time could correct Canada's Capital for "capital coveting career types"-- not even crossing their path could cease these easily greedy monetary slaves.

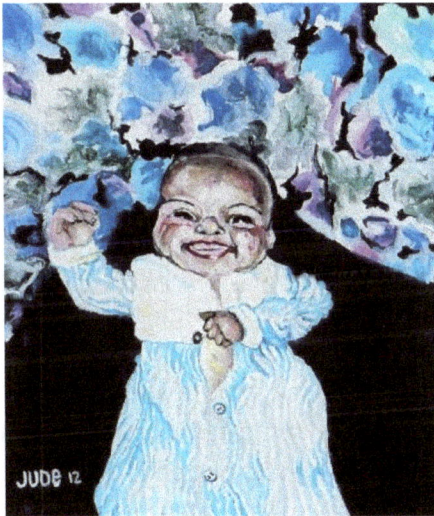

Then I was there. The longest bridge that I had ever started to cross loomed ahead. There was a sidewalk of a sort, just narrow enough to scare the crud out of me. But before embarking I was beckoned by some man seeming oddly out of place at the bridge's beginning. He offered me a way out of my courageous challenge, coercing me to enter the ravine to the side, steep and scary and reminiscent of past sexual assaults. I chose the bridge. Summoning up surreal strength, I sauntered saucily around the astonished man and began my bridge crossing event. Years later, I would reminisce of Munch and his Scream painting. I however remained silent since one specific thing I did remember was my Mom cautioning that "Ladies don't scream". You should've heard pins dropping during my giving birth of our baby girl, Amanda Mead.

It took about one hour, tight-walking between fast traffic and a vast valley where a ribbon road lay, donned-up with various vehicles full of diminutive money mongers. Did they not know they could be free like me? Having to cross the most fast and foreboding, nicely narrow road, noted for the Don Valley Parkway below, that it bridged, made me aim at success in the desire to remain on this side of Heaven.

So, after an hour, my abridged meanderings with a new anti-currency mandate had scored a few extra points, seeing the escape of rape possibilities, consequently the rank resistance of some man's lulling to a ravenous ravine...then I actually made it across this entire bridge...so that would affirmatively defer the failure to warm up in the variety store that had no compassion for me. Tallied up, my points were in the positive, I was well on my way, although not WELL enough to decipher that there was in fact a second Chinatown in a city of this size. I had imagined only one. Nevertheless, my points were positive, and I spent a moment (and inevitably some indulgence deficit) to recall the moment in Jamaica when I hopped across a tarmac to the terminal giving one last emancipated glance directly upwards to see one grey-haired amazingly supportive Rasta. HE knew. I slipped into the terminal door returning my attention to things actually below the roof of that airport. Back to reality. But I think I digress.   Back to insane, illogical adulthood as a polytechnicophrenic artist with no need, apparently for food

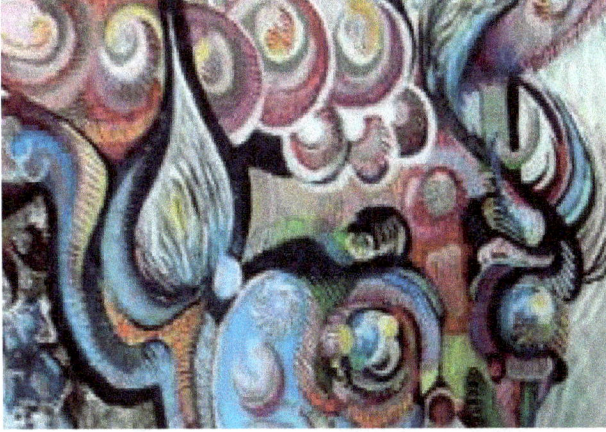

Polytechnophrenic art

(more points) or sleep (same) The bridge seemed to take about seven years to cross; I guess I really COULD stop time... just involuntarily. Man, it's cold. I need to pee. I had sat on a park bench overlooking that bridge's ending, and someone had written "Jude and "Sting", carved the summer before by someone with the name of "Jude", I surmised. Hey, I really need to pee.

Wishing that the birds had inspirational aid concerning my urinary concerns, I caught sight of eight, a good few, hurriedly hurling their feathered bodies across a road at an acute angular track and my attention returned to those stupid money-people everywhere. Hey, I actually startled this small group with my passing their pack's path trajectory. More points against money. I felt encouraged that my anti-currency stance was so successful, but somehow, my attention kept going back to toilets. Why did I leave home?   Where is home? I AM NOW HOMELESS. I really need to pee!

I traversed until the CN tower had become a toothpick with a tiny olive on it. East Toronto. I walked for four days. Yada yada. I remember walking through a memorable Armistice day ceremony.   And a parade.   Then I went too far West and

111

ended up in the Brewery district...looking up to see a digital billboard exclaiming, "Congratulations, Judy" I had really gone too far, so I headed back a bit to Yonge street. There was a humongous bookstore claiming to be the largest in the world with an ample section on the Police and the Skinhead sub culture. Hey, *I* was bald!

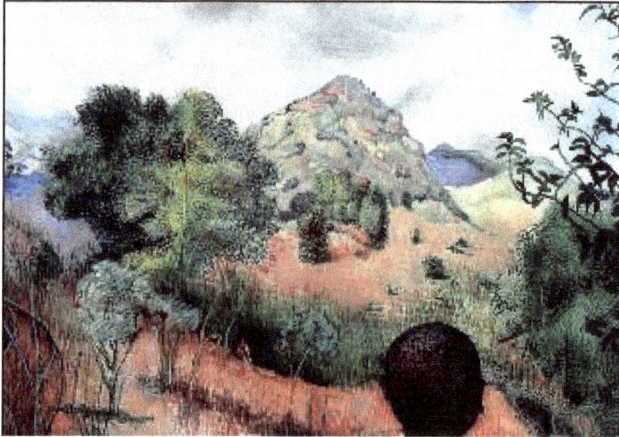

The grand spumoni mountain

I accepted both, not hesitating. But also, I discovered a place on Yonge street where I could not only pee, but have a redemptive coffee with respect as the key ingredient. Thank you, Jesus for the Huntley Street people helping the young Yonge Street street-people like me.

Now, there is some stuff to recall and also recall poorly, since I was very psychotic and sometimes under the influence of crud...just remember that I am actually reliving this as I write, and therefore words are scarce and simple. Or so I think. There was this guy who latched onto me like a malnourished pit bull, a

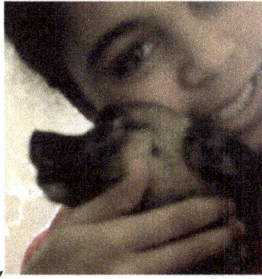

real skinny puppy, and the first time I resurfaced from my blackout (I cannot really call it a "High") he was so very relieved that I had snapped out of whatever happened. I gave him a good scare. This young man had many phobias, and since he lived near Jarvis and Yonge, he would ask me to walk him home, in the middle of the night, to avoid anyone gay molesting him. I was his bodyguard. And, so, once he was safely home, I had the sudden opportunity to walk back home for the duration of about an hour, in the night's canopy. Alone. I remember once at the corner of Yonge and Bloor, standing in wait of a green light, and a large black stretch limo creeping around that corner...me on the sidewalk waiting for that light to change.

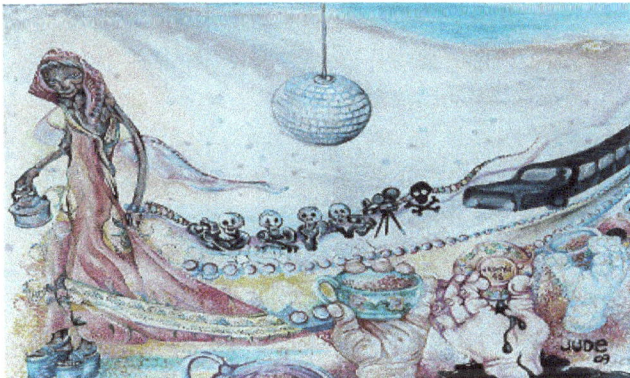

'Round the Corner Slowly

I was invisible, a true nobody. I can only imagine who was inside. It indeed could have been one of the "Big three", a trio that visited Toronto in the Autumn of 1984, causing a stir, but I, I watched their highly hyped individual descents on T.O.

from my family living room, broadcast through our floor model color television. Each time.

There was his Holiness, Pope John Paul, (the second).. Talented, Michael Jackson, (the still brown)...and Her Majesty, Queen Elizabeth, (the second). All I know was somehow I was safely in my house in Hamilton to witness the trilogy of mayhem in comfort, three times over. Over the television. Divine protection.

When Pope John Paul the Second came to T.O. town to visit, I remember that the whole place shut down. Roads, partitions, police on large horses. I meandered aimlessly from one block to another trying to find where I last left that pesky bus station, anyway. Then it happened: a black garbage bag of a hefty size was blowing across the grounds of Queen's Park... it was heading straight towards some Catholics, happy in their anticipation of fun, Their day could be ruined...not only that fact, but two police officers, laughing away could have thought that I, I was the origin of that selfsame low flying black plastic garbage bag. So I thought with stealth and grabbed that bag and, by then I was about two feet from those armed officers, so I...I...handed them that bag. They replied, can you believe it, "Thank, you, miss". So the Pope raced down the major thoroughfares of downtown Toronto, none the wiser. Not that the Pope is not wise, anyway. I had, in my wise way, rallied to catch that bus back to Hamilton, and witnessed the zooming Popemobile by floor-model color television in our living room.

Michael Jackson...left my heart broken, his story so sad. He was just beginning to suffer that horrible skin disease, his scalp burned bald in many spots, his nose too big to be a real "Jackson" family member somehow, his painful shyness, his genius...some people are born great, some achieve greatness, and some have greatness thrust upon them.

And then there is Her Majesty, The Queen. Oh well.

But there existed those few who thought me worthy of love, like the young woman in the coffee shop, desperately offering an alternative to raggedy clothes and too-small footwear and hunger that had become mania from unfed highs. She simply offered me a rose and one after another reason to accompany her to a nice place to live. With every idea I would in turn respond in the picking of a single rose petal,

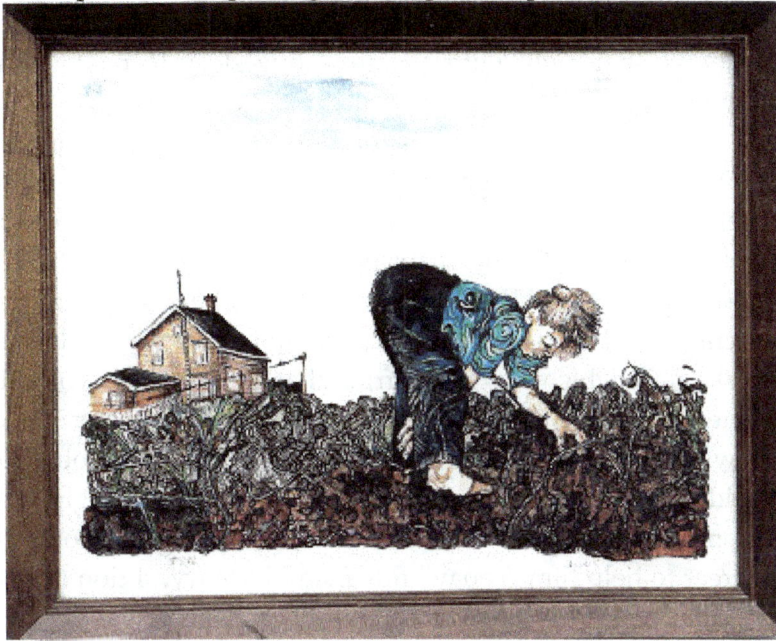

"Weeding out wrongly"

she grappling for reasons to thrive in safety, I responding with another petal picked. Finally she said "You really want to survive" and left dejected-like. I quickly went to a nearby table and successfully bummed an entire cigarette, enjoying victory.

Another episode, this same psychotic guy had me pinned against a fridge in my rooming house screaming that I was the devil. I was giddy with laughter. I do not remember how that scene ended.

So he would lead me through the streets of T.O., with his hands clasped behind him and I was to follow, so any chance I got, I detoured, albeit briefly. One night he took me and a young teen that he called Gilligan on a bus ride. I had decided that I was magical, and did not need to offer bus fare, so I merely cupped my hand over the money-receiver thing, gave the driver a knowing look and proceeded to the bus rear. The other two paid their fares and defeated my entire experiment, lacking any Faith. The bus driver told us off and demanded his due, and went home that night with an interesting story to relate to his family.

But we were on that bus for a reason, finally stepping off, I think, near Mississauga, and traversing hastily to a man's house. When we entered, our names were announced, were sat down in a basement full of mirrors, and given something like rum to sip. Our FIEND that brought us here went into an adjacent room with this man, and Gilligan and I were subjected to a fake fight which was heard from that other room beyond the basement mirrors, while we refrained from drinking our drinks. I knew their strategy and reassured Gilligan that we would not be sold, so we did not have to interrupt that false "fight over owed money" going on in jest, and end up giving our bodies to the street to help him "repay" this man. Nice try. I don't know how I disassembled that bomb, but it became an actual dud and soon we were headed back home, back to T.O. rather, by bus.

I repeated my bus fare strategy, surprised that they of little Faith still hadn't caught on. What else. What else. Oh, it might seem that I remember a remarkable amount of my psychotic days...but the fighting off of frenetic foes found me with brain damage, something mimicking being branded whilst high. I cannot explain, but these instances are tattooed.

One night, my best friend and a couple others were travelling through the subway terminal at the Eaton Center, Yonge and Dundas, in the submerged bowels of downtown Toronto, and he decided to attack someone with an exacto knife. I stopped it, incurring wrath but saving my future husband George's neck from the blade exactly near his jugular.

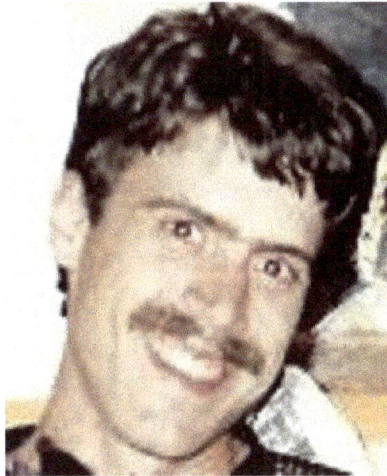

Later in life, George and I would relate memories, fragmented but for real, of the two of us meeting around downtown T.O. It was ironically synchronistic...just not in the way I had imagined the resolution unfolding. And this-this wannabe lawbreaker was having no luck. Years later I would see him on Toronto TV, a news item. It seems, he was in danger of being deported to his country of origin based on three facts: He had a prison record, he had Schizophrenia and he had Aids. I was happy to see his entire family rally to keep him here, where he could be helped the most, I must hope. This seems definitively detailed, but it has been decades of reeling under the fear I felt, and the awesome act I played, and pretended with fake calmness. Only now, under the influence of Clozapine for twenty-five years can I release these scenes from my brainscape. There is more.

There was this man that I met early on in Toronto and became friends with, and learned his story. He had worked and was fired from the electricity company by falseness rendered from the hands of his superiors. Unjustly. This man, as well as most that I met at eighteen, I remember his story more than any name. He had warned his higher-ups of a discrepancy that could have cost them millions of wasted currency. He, not a guy to shy away from conflict, fought his termination. Finally, he felt that I, having heard his story, was now able to appear before the Ombudsman, to say he was a 57 year old man, wrongfully dismissed, and proceed to relate his story. I entered the office, requested a visit, sat down, waited, and then was escorted inside the office. I hastily began my tale...of being a 57 year-old man and I had been wrongfully dismissed from my job, and had been unemployed for years working for my justice...in and out of court...I gave my personal best story. So the Ombudsman gave me a card with the name and address of a mental health clinic where I could get help. Success! I rendered this card to that man only to receive an angry response at my inaccuracy in my story— HE was the one fired from HIS job. I could not understand his non-appreciation of the sudden break in my personal rain-clouds. I could see the light. I was starting to realize...

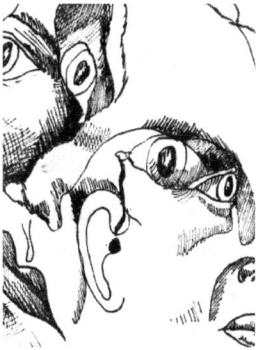

So he took me to Greek town for a buffet meal and I kept switching plates over and over as I was unable to determine which plate was poisonous. We tried a restaurant named after a skiing resort in neutral Europe and I just could not judge if Jude would, or should order the largest or the least food in the menu. My parents once arrived at my room to offer me a meal at a hamburger-joint, and I remember not quite stealing my Father's cigarette pack from their car.

Anyway, I was almost done with the T.O. leg of my walkabout and was nearly home, when I made an executive mid-street decision to free-lance what I had in my possession...me...

for forty dollars. There were these two men that I approached, sounding more homeless than street workers. The one man said, non judiciously, "Street kid", and the other one I fell in love with, remembering him from somewhere, before...however time elapses, anyway. I went away penniless but happy, having succeeded in finding my true love. Again.

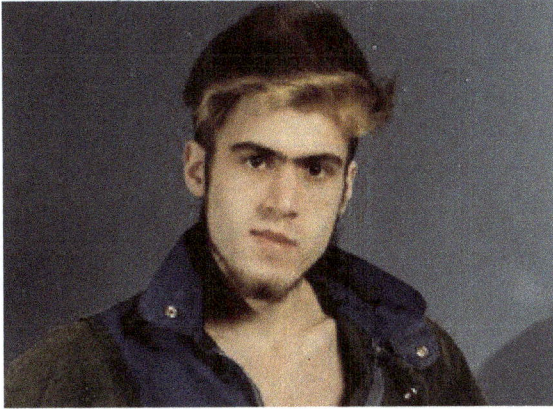

Finally finding my room once more, I had decided to forgive my parents for whatever case I had against them: trepidation ebbing the tread of my too-small runners till I was safe anew. I had learned that a hair tweezer was enough, wedged into a key point in my solid wood room door. But I was back, and my well-coiffed parental examples, Mom and Dad showed up. Having attended an awards event for successful young black adults (the irony is excruciating) and dressed to perfection. I guess mine was the after-party. I remember sitting on my trashed room floor, looking up at the two last people I would ever need forgiveness from. Or so I thought. However Jude had decided that the anger and disapproval of these now newly loved ones had been pounded out, away on the pavement. Mom said something like

"I guess we've lost a friend".

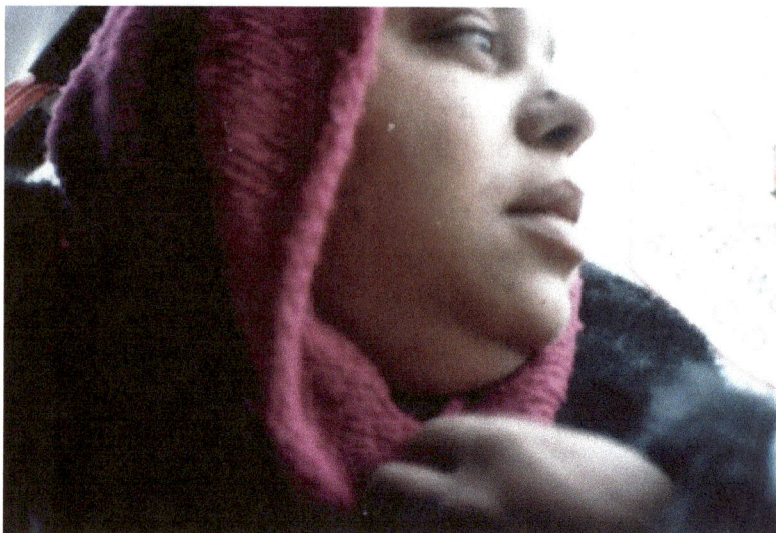

I weighed the implications of such a statement and remembered visiting a priest for Catholic confession (I being Lutheran, guys) that evening. He must have been a young priest. For my attempt at confession was full of my boasting of magical exploits, potential, not realized. And basically I scared him away. After finding out I was truthfully Lutheran, he suggested we say the" Our father"… and he cleared out, left in a flurry. Several men pointed angrily to the Church exit as I prayed after confession, and I knew, finally, that perhaps Toronto Art College was not working out for me. But as always, there was one last respite. In the immediate trajectory of their pointing toward the exit, there was this wonderful statue of Our Lady, and I

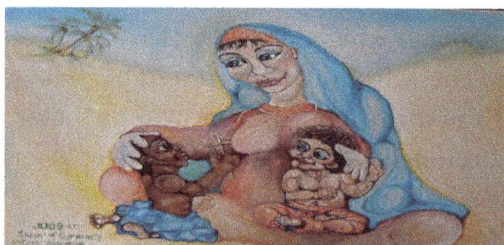

remembered years of Lenten Vespers where I loved chanting the Magnificat, in our Lutheran Church. That was it. That was "enough" of the young people who used my blackouts to their advantage. Enough of the wandering, enough of the hunger, enough of those youthful teens that insisted on mocking my bald head, enough of the cigarette butts that I would reap off the sidewalk and then ask anyone for a light, enough of the running through Chinatown, aided by removal of runners, and the not peeing... Mom then asked with impeccable timing if "I had had enough."

As we pulled away from that rooming house to head back to Hamilton, I noticed three cabbage heads, illegally picked, then discarded on the front lawn. (Bathurst and Bloor was in the midst of "CabbageTown", a place where loads of folks grow cabbage in backyard cabbage patches). I saw those cabbages as being the authentic, actual cabbage-heads known as us three, my parents and me, as we left Toronto.

The ride back to Hamilton was peaceful and eerily quiet. The lake had a November glow due to the fog hovering over it. I had prayed that the time stopping would stop soon. As I pen these words I relieve the numbness and newfound regret felt until we finally turned the highway curve and saw Coote's Paradise,

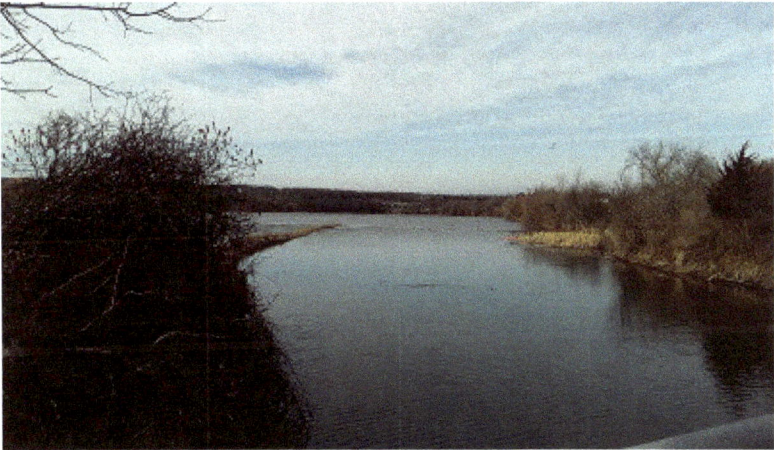

a Hamilton landmark proclaiming that this young hoot-owl had grown wise enough to appreciate a Steeltown sanctuary. There are a number of mentally ill in Hamilton, some of the lucky ones have had a similar ordeal trying hard to settle down in Toronto, the "Meeting Place" only to return to a Haven for Hell survivors. Hamilton.

Reverse Psychiatry. That is how I met my Mom

Chapter Two: Georgie

"And then, Georgie would make the fire light…"
Bob Marley

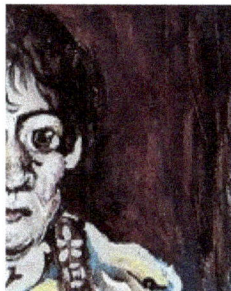

Georgie

Okay. So Bob Marley had a friend named Georgie. My older brother John would announce this FACT because it was real, to the whole of Jasmine street every morning early, blasting from his stereo speakers. Two different Georgies. One reality to shatter into two, far in the future. John was self-indoctrinated into the Reggae movement. Why not? He was also Jamaican, born biracial, intelligent, musically creative, and shared the Bible as the ultimate source of truth. Even Bob was baptized in the final chapter of his own life. John was always by heart a lover of Christ Jesus. His moment of truth boiled over one day when, finally he gave up on alternative and militant religions…albeit to a clever beat. He had played every album, probably eight, well, quite a few…at least two-hundred dozen times…it was his moment of rebellion's self-finding-out, that parsec of universal expansion, in an adolescent mind from deviation to: conformity, without losing his personal spark. I witnessed it. John asked me in a quiet minute of meaning-searching, "Do you think Hallie Selassie is God?

My immediate and undoubted response was "NO". I ensued with my theological thesis, which follows,

1. Did Hallie Selassie ever claim to be God?--No. He practiced Christianity in the Ethiopian Orthodox Church.

2. Did he die for your sins?--Negative.

3. Did he rise again?--Nope. Strike three for Selassie.

Brother John

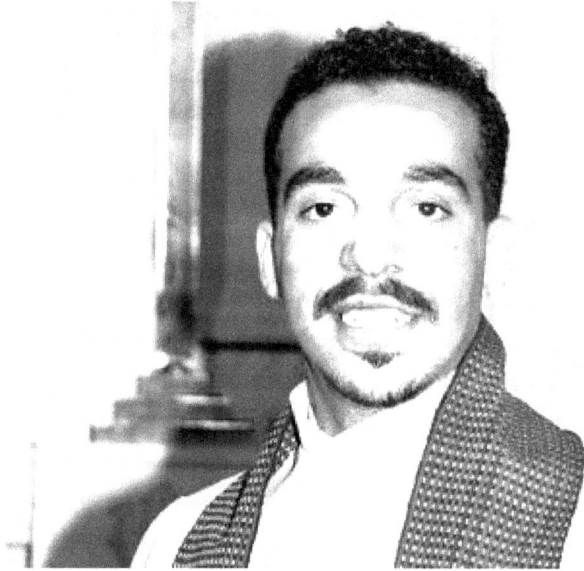

John went on to become a Minister, with two Doctorates: one earned(?) and one honorary(?). He also completed two Masters' Degrees in both Religion and Theology, trotted around the globe several times as the CEO of a Lutheran Relief Organization, and then worked as the President of a Lutheran University...all from the tender coaxing of his little sis, just newly graduating from Confirmation class. The best education I ever had. Oh, and John and Monique, his wife, both sat on a float in the Tournament of Roses Parade, for the Lutherans.

So, Georgie, the one that I personally knew in the REAL world, became my springboard back to normalcy. When I first met him we had already been living together. How's that for all you prudes or show-offs? Jude and George met about a half-day after his moving into his room, in a crucial place, a boarding house for young Schizophrenians. Oh and we BOTH had locks on our doors. I had gotten home from my job as an artist for kids, and there he was, sitting aside my place at the supper table. And there he was, smoking away in the appointed lounge. And there he was at the daily evening doughnut-eating contest at eight o'clock P.M.. after receiving bed meds. And I wouldn't see him in the morn as the norm, since he slept in.

So, as it occurred in time, I ranted about this gorgeous guy who sat aside at dinner and stole minute little glances in mid-puff, this George.

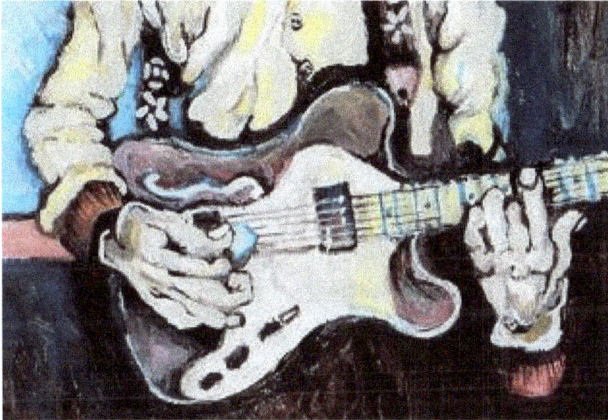

Checkout Guitar George

I was at my resident artist job at the Children's Museum, in mid-rant, when to my ecstatic discovery, someone arrived to see...me! I ran down the staircase to the gallery exhibit level to see, Georgie! He had walked about four and a half miles to my place of paltry pay for employment; from home, the boarding home, to see if he could volunteer as a guitarist. Right! I, without a word, turned and re-ascended those stairs, transcendent in emotion, forgetting to say Hi! In order to say "He's HERE!" to my co-workers' amazement. George and I ended up singing

Dinosaur songs to five year old children in fifteen minute sets, twice daily. At the time that was all we could handle.

But we both loved music. Our first official song together was "You are the sunshine of my life" by Stevie Wonder in the selfsame lounge where we smoked whilst exchanging infatuated glances.

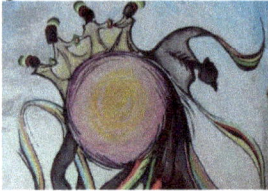

The sunshine in my life

Our second one was "That's just the way it is", a Hornsby penned protest of prejudiced preferences based on race. After those first few days, George felt the pull of former family-unit life and disappeared to play rock music with his brothers, the four of them spending days pounding away in their largish parental home. One of the times when George came back he invited me to his self same parental domicile, as well as the occasion of his brother's birthday, about a week later. So, our first date was to aim at eating lobster at a nice restaurant. George's Mom, Barb, and brother, Larry, accompanied, Afterwards, we went to the family home and enjoyed some espresso (or was it cappuccino?) and I snapped to meet his Dad. George said..."and this is my father, Guy"...I made an effort toshake his hand and discovered that Dr. Guyon Mersereau... was almost six inches less in height than George, who conversely was about half a foot taller than his Dad. I kid you not. Guy had been a pre-preparedness-era preemie, I mean, back in 1933, he had been very lucky to survive at seven month's gestation.

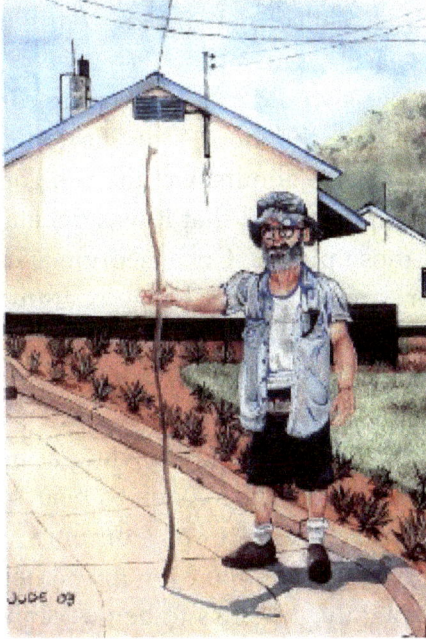

Dr. Mersereau, I presume

After that evening, I did not attend George's brother Lou's birthday celebration. It was very plain to me. George did not ask to verify our next meeting, so...I did not go. Purposely.

Our next big gig did not include myself in the least, or at least not in my bodily presence, George and Larry had rented a recording studio, with two original songs to tape. Written by Lar. They were there three days, resulting in a FANtastic demo tape. You see, there was this contest on an area radio station, and they hoped to impress someone other than the entire populace of Southern Ontario...me. What's wrong with that?

So the entire family joined ranks and collectively voted 1000 times a day, or so, to keep the Schizophoniks on top of the contest charts. Wow. I had met my own rock star and Georgeie was digging it, hopefully not to his own grave. But it gets better. They were on the top for at least three days, absolutely obliterating my obsession with Sting. For now...? I mean he could have at least called me, right? Pardon the humor, if detected.

The three of us would make the entire coffee circuit, from one Tim Horton's to the next Tim Horton's, and then the occasional Country Style donuts, we, the Schizophoniks and me, we three. We'd laugh so hard that it was debatable if we'd soon be kicked out of those places. Once Georgie and I were asked to leave simply for smoking herbal ciggys from the downtown health-food store (that only remotely smelled like pot), and actually (avoiding Jamaican shame) contained none of it at all. How soon we forget our Toronto days. But I was living hard with the Mersereaus, from ten-pin bowling at near midnight, to crashing a cavernous basement venue to hear some cover band play badly, to the prospect of camping on the family farm...which required permission from my Father.

Dad said plainly, "There's to be no Monkey business" of which I, myself responded, without thought, "Oh, Man!". Whatever happened to pragmatic silence? So we did not go. But Dad was getting tired of "Georgie Porgie monopolizing on all of your time, Judeh."

So George went to church with us.

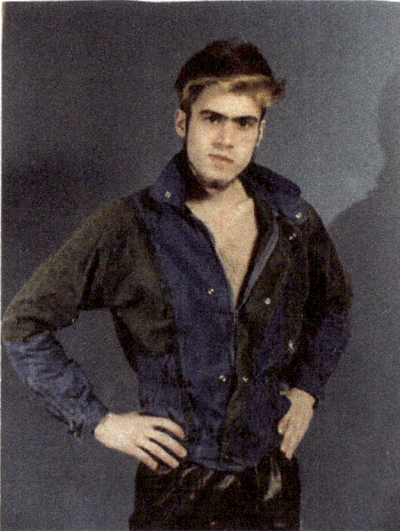

He also sang in the choir. And when his best friend, let's call him Rob Chapman, informed me of a series of unfortunate happenings to my Georgie, I was convinced. Overlooking that we had dated for nine full months...without even kissing. Man, we were infatuated. So I endeavored to stipulate that George must have an interest in God, or all deals were off. Things went downhill from that instant, as George proposed marriage at a friendly Country Music bar, on a whim of jealousy...there were semi-drunken revelers present and you can guess my response. Sure! You can believe it, I assented, impressed with his choice in women. Soon after, it happened. We kissed for the first time, George expressing ultimate Yang-ness.

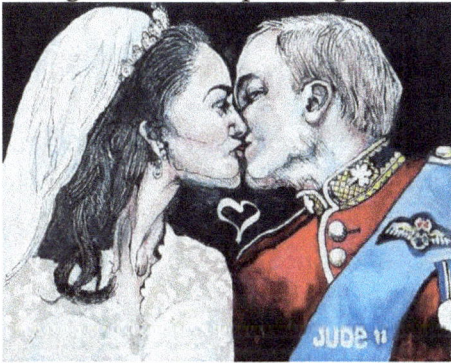

So I moved out of that boarding house to reside at our family home...and of course as a year-long protest, worked at McDonalds for one year to the day. Because my art would not sell.

I deduced that George and I were not to marry. Since I really wanted to be a Catholic nun. Figure that one out. The mind of a newly recovering schizophrenian is hard to understand even by themselves. I remained a heavy smoker, whilst buying up all the Catholic literature I could find. I attempted the rosary every night, not getting far... I guess my math had abated over the years.

So Georgie was actively and purposely abhorred for eight long lunar cycles on the understanding that he was on pot and also denied being a skinny money person. I practiced non-prompted disgust. I lowered my medication. I earned employee of the month. I got engaged to a nice man, Catholic and willing to live as Priest and Nun. I rejected the same poor guy upon our first kiss...stating that it had reminded me of George...somehow myself and this Man, whose only error was that he'd neglected to be George, did not last a month. Rationalizations labored on. But why George, Lord?

It seemed evident that I had forgotten that eventful afternoon after school, About four years before my own private breakup of the century from George, whilst I witnessed a local video show... showing, of all people, Sting...and he was mad and deadly serious peering through the t.v. that my Dad had bought for the purpose of respite. What did I ever do? I took that look seriously as though it was meant for none other. I mean no-one else was in the room! The video bothered suggestible me, but God always provides a way out, which I did not take initially...The Lord told me to look past that television that sat on the floor, towards the window, and onto the street. So in a breath I took a look.

I saw a young couple walking so slowly; was it a funeral? The young man wearing leather clogs and an African shirt

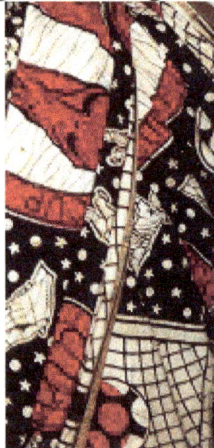

with faded bell-bottomed jeans and having hair past his shoulders, and smoking!...and this was 1983! And THIS was my chosen lover! God proceeded to tell me that I was to wed this specimen and I chimed- in my quick, "You've got to be kidding, Lord!" knee-jerk response. It did not bother me that I was conversing with God Himself...but rather that my future mate was a sixties rock relic. As soon as possible I rejected a voice from my forever Lord God about my forever love, George, and immediately was my fast reaction... that this televised rant aimed at the camera was truly "real" Right. It would be only one single moment of truth in my short life, claiming a deluded future over a Gift offered so redemptively. I had a single-cell detonation, and chose Sting. He would dominate my escalation to insanity, the product of simple protestation against the introduction of Georgie into my young life and I got sicker and sicker. After all, I was still only sixteen and more into creative exits than truthful establishments of fact. I still had cleverness under my belt. And naivety as my main defect.

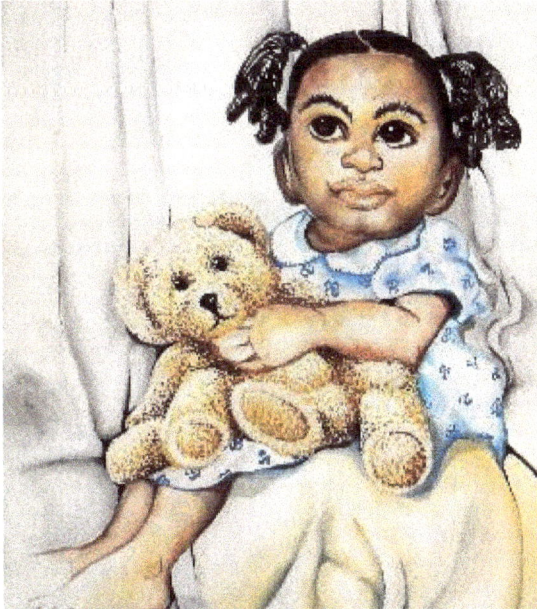

Naomi...aged three-ish

It's funny how once you learn to go with "the flow", though, you can suddenly decipher what is real either by a lucky guess, or time- aged wisdom, or from well-honed logic, or by a voice from God. Whichever is hardest to adopt.

In fact I could have remembered how (by fortune) my Father and I had given consent to allow the establishment of a boarding house down the street...those campaigning folks needed a neighborhood consensus...to (wisely) allow housing for unfortunates like that very selfsame hippie-couple in question. I entered my personal prematurely (illogical) alternate reality instead of endearing the simply ultimate guy for me (according to my personal still small voice) from Heaven's gentle prodings.

Or I could have recalled my own testimony of future spouses given to my own Dad in a much stronger way than letting George move down the street. My Father was highly intelligent and understood the minds of child prodigies, so whilst we traveled down the QEW Niagara-bound, to receive his master's certificate in Special Ed from Niagara University, I decided it was time to reveal my future husband to my Father. So I advised him to exit that highway at the next off-ramp...was it Fruitland road or Vineland road?

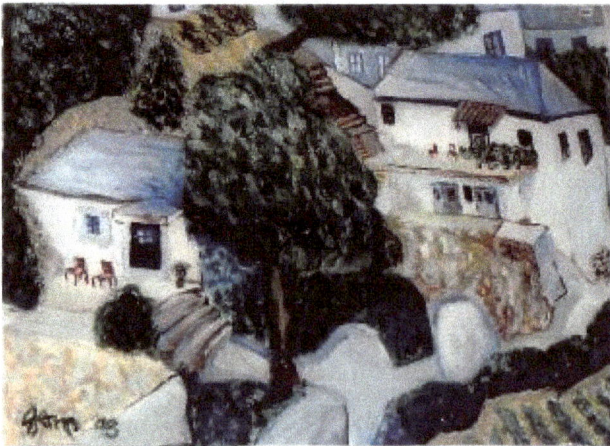

I cannot remember every little thing, you know! Anyway, there were these four wild long-haired boys in the back of a mustard colored VW van selling vine-fruits...grapes (at a tremendous profit)...And I had my choice of the four. Dad immediately warned me of the curly-haired one, and I almost chose the blonde one, but by this time, my Dad and Dr. Mersereau were shaking hands and promising to see each other at the wedding. True story. Probably lost to antiquity. But not me.

Back to the boarding home that we two had shared. George had moved away too, to an alley basement bachelor apartment, and my own self continued a herculean effort aimed at hate. Hate. Hate. This was my most successful time emotionally since mono did me in, and all I did was hate. My co-worker-slaves would ask if we indeed were in Hell...Hell wasn't this bad, I whispered back in hushed haste. Some shifts were like an acid trip, something I had never voluntarily taken, but who knew?

One day I definitely plopped a metal tray into another of comparable size that was just sitting there half-full of melted bacon fat which splashed on my upper leg. Screaming followed. The owner of this McDonald's, who was a born again Christian prayed without hesitation in a circle consisting of me and her secretaries. They then took me to the nearest emergency room, where the staff found... no burns at all. The managers of this restaurant said I was very close to understanding...which I didn't quite understand.

So somehow I was immersed in my wonderful burger patty flipping occupation, mindlessly occupying my waking hours (I slept around the clock otherwise). It kept me busy enough to earn a whole heap of money, and as my mental health waned away I was appointed dish washing as a last resort in my personal aforementioned perdition. Anyway, I quit in tears on my first year anniversary, before they got the guts to fire me, seeing that I was previously disabled, hence not to be blamed for a disabled breakdown. Right. And that they could be blamed for ruthlessness upon termination of employment.

Next step-finding somewhere to NOT be homeless. Not again. I had attended a CAT scan appointment for mental research at Mac (McMaster University Research) (McMaster not being a pun) the same day which I'd left home, for the last time, right before I abandoned my McOccupation. Mom and I had had a hapless argument which somehow landed me in...another boarding house, paying for one single night with the CAT scan stipend. (A reward for motionless good-scan behavior.) What a coincidence! AND George mulled around in his alleyway basement bachelor apartment, approximately one full block away. What!

It was fate reviving faith for both of us. One business day before I moved away to my new boarding house, that was the day that George had gotten his divorce from his first wife, the girl doddling with him in the unheard dirge down my street to the selfsame boarding house that Dad and I consented to exist. Friday walking papers...Monday Re-institutionalisation in a room. Quel coincidence!--I thought I would write it in French this time to avoid unnecessary repetition. There's more.

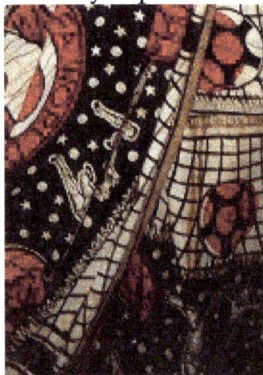

I actually ran into Georgie at a cigarette store, buying myself a number of cartons, when amazingly I heard a long unheard voice (of the real kind), and it said "Hi, Judy"

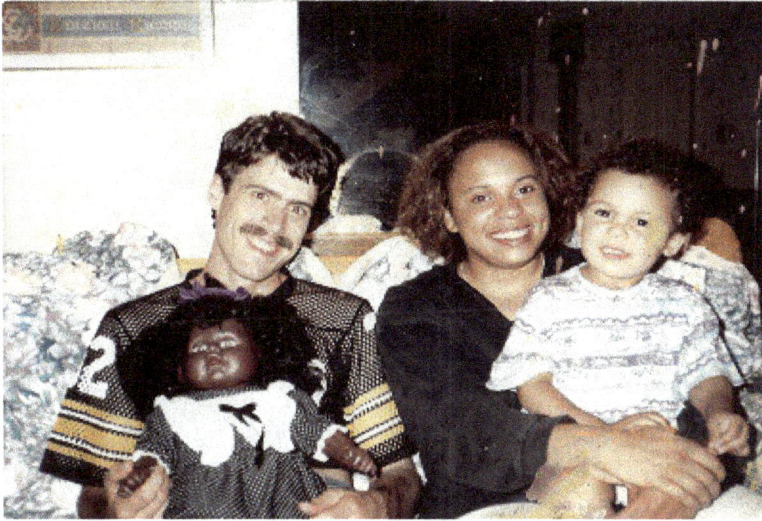

"

"The Happy family"--Brenna

We were back. And Georgie always had a light for my smokes. He mindlessly, and in the absence of me, planted about fifty books of matches in his tiny apartment in hopes of always providing an initial puff for myself and my favorite brand of cancer sticks.

Infatuation reinstalled, normal recovery in fast track, medications restored to full titration, resumed fascination, abundant matches and nothing in the delaying of marriage, which we rushed into, at an extreme velocity. I had earned and saved about 800 dollars which was enough to pay for a ceremony at the Hess Street Chapel, named after Hess Street Village in which this chapel sat. See what I mean? Potentialities were exponential.   My family in denial, Georgie's delighted, we spurred on ahead to our dream bliss and a baby! Could we care for a baby based on our caring for each other? That was to be seen.

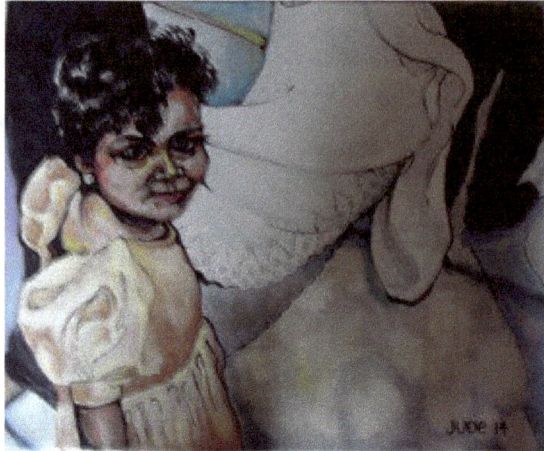

The flower girl

But first things first. My family tearfully attended our spartan nuptial ceremony...sobbing and ready to
murder, I recall. George was militantly in love and did not care...and my love was a great"ditto" in echo. There are no photos of my side of the family from our wedding day, they simply went straight home. Had I done my homework on the seriousness of entering a marital contract, I probably would have...done the same exact thing. Nonetheless, by the time nine-thirty rolled around, I was tired and weary from the most silent reception in history. If it were not for (once more) the presence of live rock music, we would have been dejected. But Larry had written a beautiful song in our honor, and George and I delivered a rousing rendering of "No woman, no cry" for our guests' tear welling eyes. So we went on to the hotel, and the first thing done was a hasty phone call to Dad to ask his blessing. He responded, as always, with affirmation and said "I was at your wedding, wasn't I?" By the way, for you young ones, the marriage starts the MOMENT you complete your vows, not after the honeymoon is one month over. We tried to stay up all night, and ordered about four carafes of coffee. Had room service not closed for the night, we would probably have beaten the wedding-night.

The marriage ensued... However I had a sneaking suspicion that I had married for money. After a year at McDonald's. I mean, really. After all, I had lost weight too, right? George, ever in love, responded that he also had married for money, calling to mind the 800 or so dollars that I had saved from my McJob, had I not spent the bulk of it on the wedding itself, which actually was quite magnanimous on my part, apparently...so, we were even. But as a direct repercussion, I had the post wedding willies of being a greedy one. This lasted for approximately thirty years. We just celebrated our thirty-first anniversary. I think the two of us are finally safe and in the clear. For now.

"I remember..."   --Bob Marley

Chapter Three:

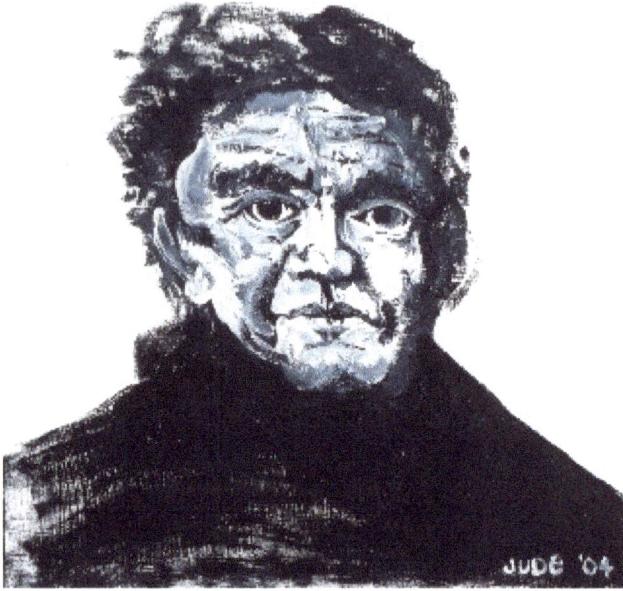

1
"We got married in a fever..."

Johnny and June Carter Cash

Thank God for country music. Not only is it hard to understand why one would utter such singing sounds but it is equally difficult to decode those words. But wonderfully for the two of us, country was advantageous. There was this song, "forever and ever, Amen" which said it all. Back with a vengeance, although I really never should have reduced my medication, for it was what I fell back on without George to focus on fixated-like. So Sting made a reappearance in my head, and apparently nobody else could notice the entrance of Georgie's upstaging understudy. Just me.

Might I add that whenever I waxed reluctant to take my meds...like when I had my pregnancy with Amanda, our baby, the resident Angel in the entire family's collective agreement by far, well, Sting would reappear. I was pregnant within a couple of months after marrying, our girl-child being born on Brother John's birthday. Which was cool. My Psychiatrist had given me the choice of taking my psych medication and possibly hurting the unborn one, or continuing smoking as a coping mechanism during gestation. I chose to smoke, and had a complete psychotic relapse by the pregnancy's ending.

Eighteen hours and one half of labor accompanied with the erupting voices. When twelve hours had elapsed, I felt timing was appropriate to calmly suggest an epidural for pain. I remember the Resident Doctor saying, "try to show a little restraint" to her own protege taking mental notes...but this had been nine long months, the baby 9 days late, and half a complete day of not pushing, and I really thought the doctor was talking to ME. I got my epidural. It stung. Then I heard a voice saying, "that's one more dead N....", (not Nunes) so I decided to arch my back, needle in place, to see the doctor who'd declared me deceased. We were introduced...some moments are lost in antiquity. Although this moment of truth still might qualify on Judgment Day. Still after that, I was told to simply not push as three or four other babies were delivered in the interim.

But our time came at the darkest hour, and I and George pushed for an hour and one half one, and I, recalling our prenatal lessons' predictions, announced something irrational to show I was delirious during labor and said,"I LOVE GREEN", an out-and-out lie: I hated green, but at least it proved everything was textbook congruent. Finally Dr. Sargent, (Seriously?), gave the orders to not push until he got this Suction-Cup thing to "kiss" Amanda's head and pull her out. While his back was turned, I realized the absurdity, and gave one decisive final push, and Amanda was born, flying onto this awaiting table, with a scream at a comedic pitch emanating from her healthy lungs, which made me laugh, and then I noticed...there were about seven professionals in the room, and a preemie incubator...they all had thought that she would not be alright, but a Mother knows.

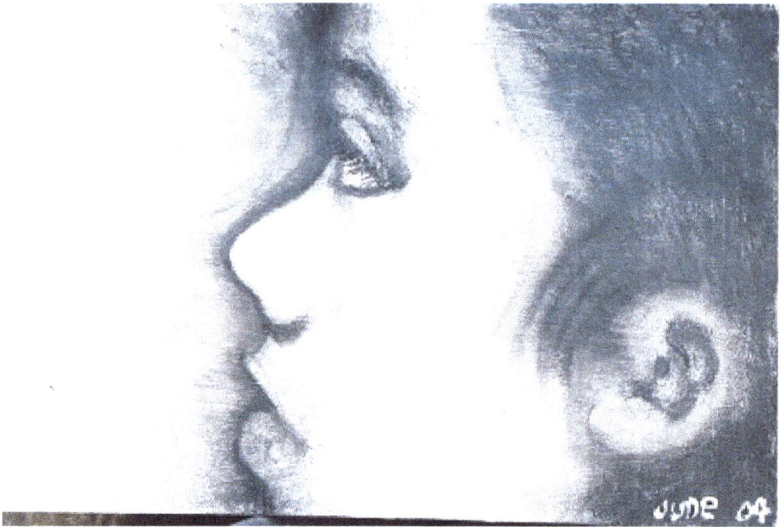

I cried, exuberant, as Georgie had returned from a cigarette break to hold his daughter in tears of Fatherly love regarding the most beautiful thing he had ever seen. Amanda Mead.

Amanda means "lovable" and Mead means "honey".

Maybe, everybody, now is an opportunity to describe my return to breakdown-mode since Manda was born. Despite the world-wide happy occasions, such as the fall of the Berlin wall, the fall of Soviet Communism, the success of Dan Hill's song about an unborn heart, the freeing of Nelson Mandela from a lengthy prison sentence, and the (almost) freeing of China, simple fragile Jude slipped once again into insanity. My Dad had called me one Sunday morn to announce to the "Nowhere Girl" that jubilant South Africa was celebrating the liberation of Mandela with the words, "Amandla Mandela. The only problem was Dad, now called Papa, altered that exclamation by stating maniacally the concept that they were really chanting, "AMANDA Mandela".

What was worse, my Public Health Nurse was presently visiting...a house call on a Sunday morn?...and in conversation slipped the fact out that she originated from South Africa, the land of Mandela. And then suddenly, my Case manager was there, her face made to look like various veggies, a carrot for a nose, cucumber eyes, ruby red-pepper hot lips, maybe mushrooms for ears, and suddenly my Psychiatrist appeared to be appalled that one of my male former friends had become a nymphomaniac, even though he claimed to be of the male race. Hospitalization City. I had in truth exhausted my own self with around the clock feedings, cleaning, sleeping, sleeping some more, smoking, sweeping, changing diapers, making up bottles in advance, I was the true vegetable, and was admitted to the Hospital, asap.

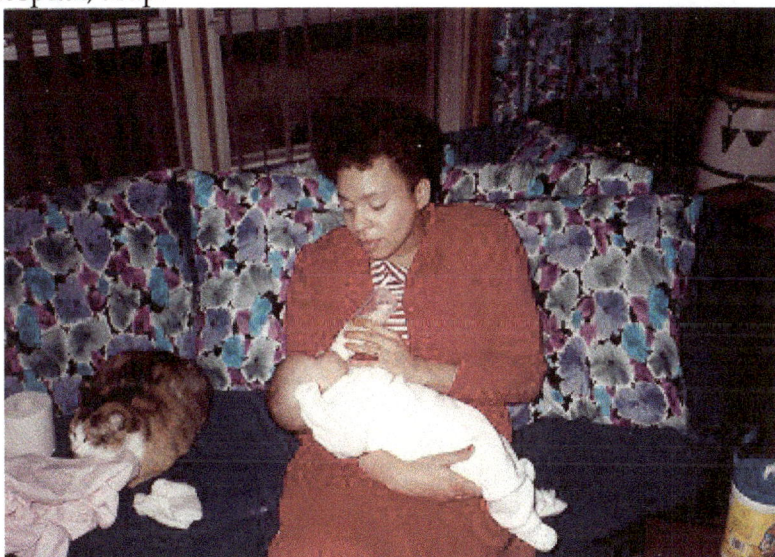

Trying my hand

They put me in seclusion so that I could sleep, and all I could hear were the near to nursing station doors slamming, slamming, my doors of opportunity, slamming shut a hundred times an hour. Because I had kept my baby. No music fame. No modeling. Incoherent babbling art. The doors kept slamming and I kept failing to keep my food down, exhausted. It seemed like plastic sustenance anyway. And then it happened. Our collective family stepped in! I remember that night when all involved directly declared that they would gladly live from crisis to new crises. The world's best family, merely.

A true miracle. We could not take care of little Amanda, but our families granted us the honor of seeing her whenever possible, not even litigating any terms or conditions. She thrived and was fought over by George's three brothers as to who was the "Fun Uncle". A dozen stuffed monkeys surfaced, each called after something healthy to ingest. Like Burdock, or Dikon. She grew cuter and probably could have died from Acute Cuteness. Not one of us worried, since she was our miracle babe.

Brenna, (spelled correctly), my only sister, eternally good with young ones, became a Godmother, and to this date has never caused me, or Amanda grief. Blessings increased in multiplicity. And we, now Jeordy, never stopped trying to have our baby beauty full-time. Ever. Not even when she moved out at seventeen years old.

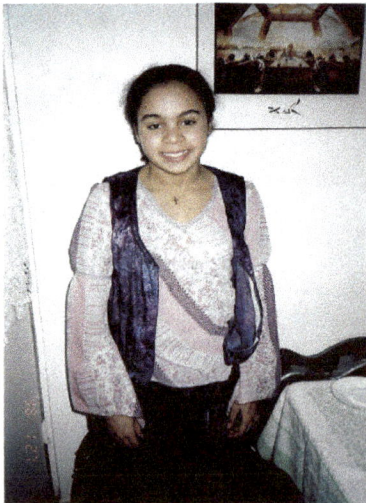

Manda's Confir-
Mitzvah

We could not shoulder the workload of caring for Manda, but we cared for her without wavering. We took her to Suzuki violin classes, with submarine sandwiches to sink afterwards. We waited for her school bus from Hillfield Strathallan College, where she was enrolled in the only PART time, although

Montessori, vacancy in town. Then it was grade school. At her first day's computer class, the teacher requested that a sentence would be attempted to be written...our child wrote a paragraph, unearthing covert genius, and not surprising any of her family contingent. We waited for her emergence after school almost every day. She would come running and I would throw my arms out, and then she would jump, almost knocking me over. Every single day. And the other parents never laughed, not ever.

She was also kind.

We all recall calling her "The loving baby" as she handed over her supper, piece by peaceful offerings, to which we chimed, "YOU eat it". She relented, cherished and made all in the family joyful. Broccoli being her favorite food, gulped down with some pastene pasta.

She was also funny.

When I visited her school for Parent Night, It was opportune to read one of her penciled poems, and it followed,

> IN AIRPORTS you are RUSHED
> IN AIRPORTS you are HUSHED
> HUSHED, RUSHED
> RUSHED, HUSHED,
> Oh, it's all the SAME!

We laughed so hard, we two, that we thought we would be kicked out of that school. Nobody else found the humor hiding therein that peculiar poetry.

She was also innocent. Her understanding of Hide and Seek was that she would direct to the hiders exactly where to hide, and then she would count.

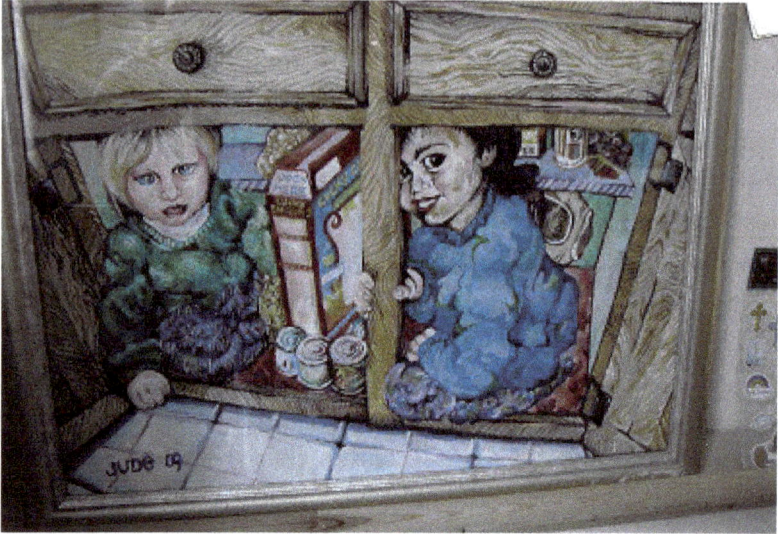

Hide-and-Seek

At night she had a mattress on the floor to sleep on (NOT a repeat of Toronto) so she wouldn't roll off too far. But never thought she could get up in the morning by herself. Instead yelling out "Mummy...Up!" every morn, especially if we were in earshot. Sometimes we stayed elsewhere, away from her, you see. Until she was three, this was the custom each morning. Every Sunday, Manda reclined in her car seat removable cradle part, She did not make a sound...actually, I do not remember her even spitting up, or suffering a diaper rash even.

Our favorite progeny, our only one, was a talented little thing. She starred in a short film, created by Kathleen Cummins, called "Emer, Banished to the waves of the sea"...I hope I've got that right.

When Amanda returned from the primary city park in our metropolis of maladjustment and misfits, Gramma Nunes asked her what went down. "We played, we went in the sprinkler, we chased squirrels"...you get the idea. Inquired of mummy..."Mummy smoked!"...Out of the mouths of babes.

When the time came, (when we two "grownups" were

ready), Georgie and I would take her to Muskoka or just slightly south of Algonquin park in the Haliburton area for the bulk of March break, by bus. Snowshoeing, swimming (indoors), jumping on the bed, and the most delish venison or salmon with red wine that you could find. These were year-round family resorts, at the far end of a seven hour bus trek. Every moment was family fun. Amanda was approximately seven years and George and I, we were almost fully mature when those trips were initiated. We swam more than once a day, at times. We had fries in a roadhouse style restaurant, which proudly displayed high up in the corner of the room...an empty bottle, devoid of beer, drunk by Mike Myers. We went for several installments of family memories during the March breaks, always successful in our return. Returning to the smoggy air around our hometown, afforded the most relieved sigh of success for us. Smog-breathed coughing would ensue eventually, of course. But it was not bad, succeeding for the first five times in a long while at something that truly mattered to us. Nuclear family vacationing.

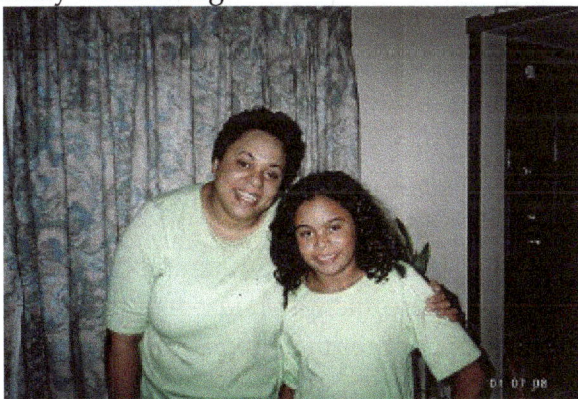

Which is the Mummy?

But what of failure? The walk to Gramma 'N' Grampa's home was a good seven blocks from our high-rise, and we must have walked it a hundred times over the years, but early on, I made a big mistake. There was this rental house along one of the "safe" side streets, where it's occupant owned several

Rottweilers. I let myself relax for one split second while the house screen door opened...we were just arriving at that part of the sidewalk as four dogs, one fully grown and three mostly mature, bounded out to the front yard. I knew what I was to do but was negligent in training Mandamead to cross her arms across her body. Well, she was bitten a few times as the owner of these monsters cursed and immediately announced the wonderful fact of his lovely pets' having their rabies shots a week earlier.

Yay.

This man offered to give us a ride to emergency, and we accepted. Five hours later, there were six(?) painful stitches in her skin and I had not left her side once. Except to pee. This time I was allowed to use the facilities. Manda being so young squeezed my hand at my prompting whenever it really hurt, to watch and feel those stitches. My sole sister Brenna arrived to support when I quite suddenly realized that I was a heavy smoker. Not bad damage control. You win some...you do the math. We litigated, so this guy got a five-hundred dollar fine, and volunteer hours, but the dogs were permitted to live. The judge noted for the record that Me and Amanda both smiled at the sparing of the Rottweilers. I guess the owner could *rot while her* stitches disintegrated away.

But we never relented in our dream of being a full time family.

Regretfully Jeordy had a roaming streak and so we moved around from apartment to house to a smelly dive above a fish and chips place...but ultimately our best stint was at a huge apartment building, sixteen floors high, where we decided to abide for a fantastic fourteen years, and a half one.

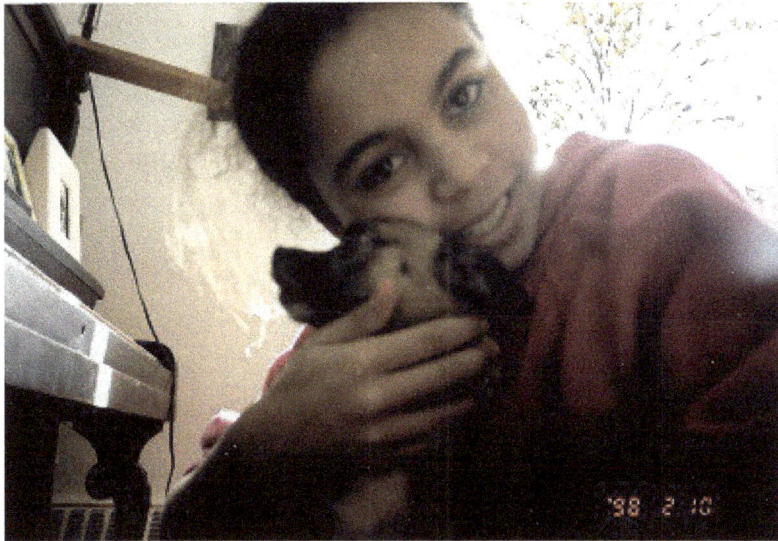

Chico Bandito

This is where we hosted Amanda increasingly often, got a tiny Chihuahua to walk (and carry his stuff on his behalf), swam in the apartment pool, played basketball at a neighboring school, and officially broke the trespassing laws in the Regional Principality of Hamilton-Wentworth.

Manda was a talented B-ball player but failed to make the ninth grade effort turn into membership on the team. So we reminded her that Michael Jordan did not make his freshman team, in his freshman year. She had known this encouraging fact, and stayed the "court course" until she was the top player. Speaking of playing, she had performed at one of the most fancy banquet halls in Hamilton many times with her Suzuki comrades, even making a tour to Newfoundland with her orchestral young buddies.

Our beloved daughter had so many friends, socialization being sooo important to potentially mentally ill ones, that we really did not worry about her developing Schizophrenia. And there was the Cleghorn clinic. Early high risk intervention, at fifteen, reassuring all involved that she would be fine. So I finally relaxed in the knowledge that there were no looming mental Rottweilers in her future. Amanda grew up so quickly after that mental examination...I had become so numb. Apparently life at any one of her homes had become unbearable, so she left and I had no "Amanda" wind in my sails.

Chapter Four:

"We didn't start the fire...

--Billy Joel

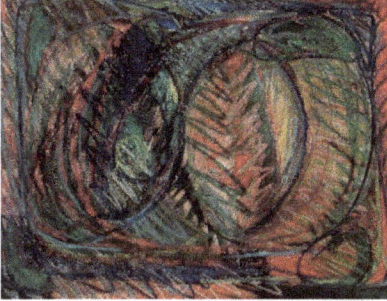

A fire

O.K. Just a little departure from former frozen times and moving in a zip from the Post Partum Psychosis Blues, and onwards. Watching television from my lounge of a different Hospital locale from fourth floor Psych, I witnessed in horror a fire that was started by some teens (Some like it hot, some...freeze as teens). It was on the premises of a tire pile reaching into the ten thousands, that burned for one month. There was no premise of such a large blaze, but others followed. I guess there are more than a couple car tire hoarders. Firefighters fought it around the clock. I thought I was the one who started it, although I had no proof against me, and was also currently on a mental Hospital ward receiving a re-installment of medications for my hopefully hasty recovery. Let's say my illness lingered longer than a few tire fires, or one immense one, however you grow tired of counting tires.

Soon after, the entire family Mersereau decided to fly collectively to Vancouver to visit brother Jack. In a plane. It seemed much harder than Jack visiting us, so we went anyway. Amanda was five months old and a true beaut. She was the most gentle, calm and aware five-month-old that could be, in the arms of other loved ones, as George and I tried to stay awake while we toured B.C. I do, in keeping with the theme of this chapter, remember surfacing to consciousness in plenty of time to see fire ravaged sticks of trees spread over many hectares. There had been a forest fire a full twenty years or more before. The trees had not remembered to be reborn. Horrific.

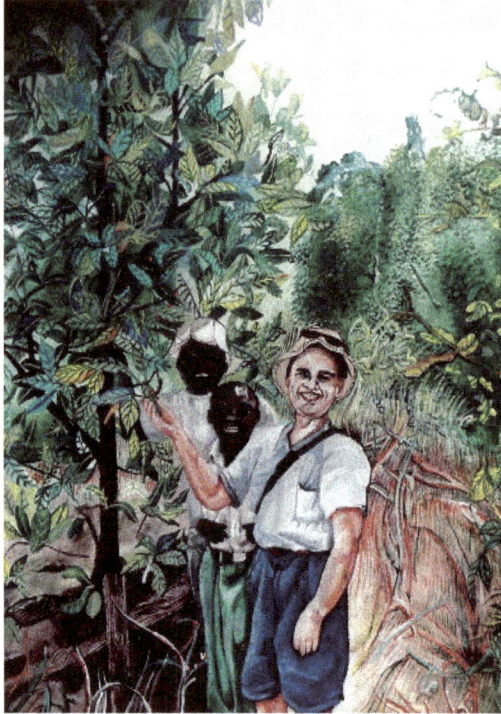

Bountiful growth

We then found this cute house that foreshadowed the tiny home craze, a luscious compact two-bedroom dollhouse. It was bliss. We signed the "lease", probably fifty one pages then assumed that it was a rent to own wonderful opportunity. Wonder what happened.   We ended up performing most maintenance duties, planting in the garden, painting the foundation concrete bricks, putting a hose to the durable and appealing plastic white siding, interiour decorating. There just happened to be a posse of teenagers who latched onto the habit of setting alleyway buildings afire in the still of the night after

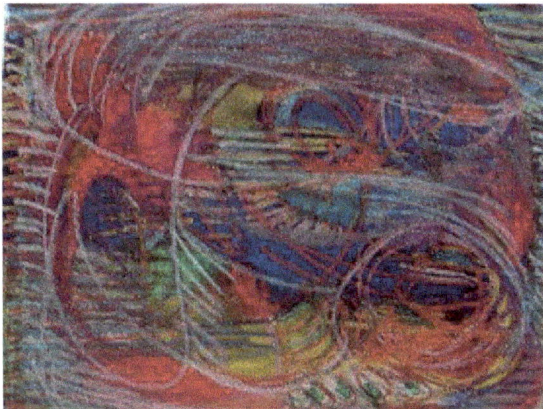

night...My nerves were shot since I had adopted the practice of staying up 'till two thirty. That was what the officials said would be the cutting-off point of the offenders' offending for the night in question. To heighten the suspense, I had been on a medication change. This was a new drug, supposed to help with psychosis, but did not. Not forever, anyway. I was paging through the dictionary in wonderment at the morphing of words, into words that never existed before, or were they from some dead language like Catalan, or Swine Latin, or some other, I could not understand yet was amazed. Then I was putting, or

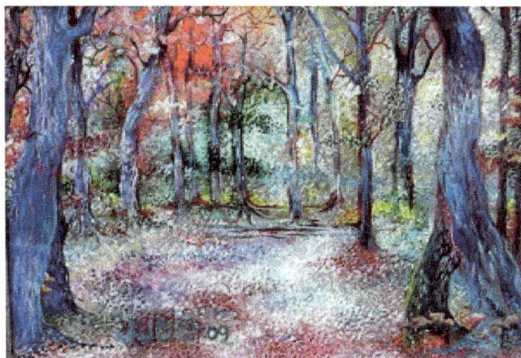

trying to, my tongue on the stove burner (Hey, an almost—fire!) because I felt I was swearing too much. I never swear. Then I put some pig statues in the cellar to ward off witches and, of course managed to attempt shaving my cat's head to further procure protection from skinheads.

The Police were surprised that someone so sick had called, welcomed them and then told her diagnosis with accuracy, hoping that they would take her to the Hospital. But that was me, forever in side-by-side worlds. One real, one not so real.

There's a place, nicknamed "The United Nations", in downtown Hamilton, a subsidized 26 floor monstrosity, housing many immigrant families of untold numbers...an apartment apart from normal apartment standards. We lived there, maintaining our own familial hopes forever and forever. The only problem was that there were alarm-happy teens who pulled the alarm nearly every night. Fire responders would arrive each time to terrorize poor Manda out of some kind of sleep patterns, ever.

So THAT didn't work. By the time a real fire, not at all serious, broke out...WE were toast.

In step with incessant effort, we then discovered the apartment, once more where we spent almost fifteen years. There was a fire there, also, a deliberate one in one of the elevators. Some people got out...some safely slept through until the morning. It was a cold night and so the Hamilton Street Railway provided a couple of buses for our comfort, the ones who had awoken. Nobody was hurt, but the three elevators were now only two fully equipped lifts.

However, these were the golden years of our little family with countless memories of ordering pizza specifically with one piece missing, scotch taping comments on the wall of Mummy's tentacles and suction cups, Ovaltine "leathers" made with the popular powder, eggs and orange juice—made by Manda and therefore ultimately delicious; and then our Chihuahua, Chico Bandito.

What can we say about Chico? Our tiniest habitual yapping artist would proliferate incessantly at his favorite activity...barking. In fact by the time that his previous owners made off with our 200 dollars, Chico displayed his own canine skills...for about an hour. He barked and barked until I had the timely realization that Chico was now mine. So, as before, I decided that we all should get along with each other and successfully broke through the initial harshness. After all, we had no inkling as to how long Chico would be ours. About seventeen years later we drove our Chico, whimpering in fear to this place. He was blind and deaf and incontinent and I could have loved to keep him here longer, but it would not be fair to him. I clumsily gave her the dog carrier, and she brought it back horribly empty. A man had just arrived at this place with his pet. He proceeded to comfort with the undeniable fact that it does not get any easier with however many pets you put down.

George's parents, one time, arrived home after a trip somewhere, when we all were apparently much, much younger, so we decided to have a little fire burning in their hearth upon entering their home. Now, for your information, there is a thing called a "flue". This had not been deployed previous to our hopeful lighting up the domicile--with warmth. The smoke, returning from halfway up the chimney caused untold billows, naturally, only not outside the chimney-top where it should be...but collecting in the house interior instead. So we opened as many windows and doors as possible. They arrived home, alright, to a cold smoke filled house and silly, guilty smiles from us three.

Then there was the Plastimet Inferno. Hamilton was a highly industrial town, having many varied companies, apart from the notorious steel manufacturers, such as the Plastimet plastics gatherers. Well, it happened that they had a fire one day. It lasted well into the night. The cloud plumes could be seen for miles, all black and definitely toxic. People from that North-end neighborhood gathered around as though it were more akin to a bonfire, hence not really rendered as fatally dangerous by those who inhaled its reeking by-products. Untold new kinds of chemicals, magic and mutant plastics to kill off more than a few of the observers, mind you, not immediately. Not just creating COPD or asthma...or something worse. Today, the Plastimet fire is rarely talked about, especially by those who have passed on.

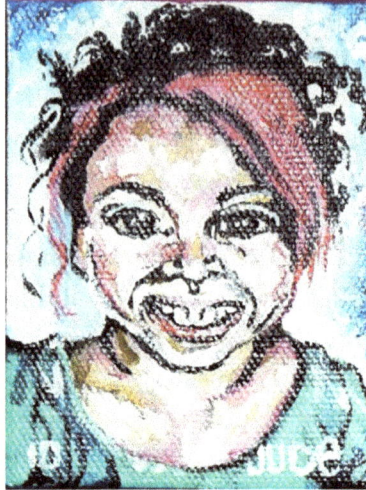

Fiery Hairdo

Our next tale of burning was a fire in our hearts. Amanda having moved on, George and I adopted the savings of our Church, St. Giles, and moved ourselves right into the neighborhood. The people that existed in the higher-ups apparently had forgotten of Jesus' saving power. This entire friendly community, really, was on the chopping block, and so we returned to George's basement bachelor alleyway apartment's building, rebuilt in the aftermath of a meth-lab explosion that blew off the roof, which erupted from George's exact former bachelor pad, in that alleyway basement. A woman and her daughter died there, and so that unit was permanently sealed closed.

So we did our best to rescue our beloved church from the narthex-nemesis and save that special sanctuary because such an incredulous indiscretion well underway would affect blocks of poorer types in the surrounding neighborhood. There was AA, for those suffering alcoholism, CA for cocaine slaves, The Elizabeth Fry association for women in a situation, a Parish

Health Nurse, pursuant health fairs, The Sherman Hub meetings, also a group that cared for those in Special Care Lodging Homes, the Downstairs Kitchen-with its' once monthly meals and constant catering for various ventures at city-wide venues, the Steeltown Symphony orchestra performances, Dance lessons, Choirs, both senior and some junior, a Deaf Ministry in case you hadn't heard, Cabaret nights, fashion shows, Turkey dinners at thanksgiving and Christmas and Easter...so they closed St. Giles United Church with some disagreement, and I was personally considered to be trouble...well, I DID suggest that they consider what God thought about this whole mess...and grew more courageous at succeeding meetings...they didn't like that. They didn't like that. One Sunday Georgie and I finished singing and playing for a contemporary service, and were flatly informed that that was the final service for St Giles, and were given a goodbye wish. We never gave up on keeping that church going.

St Giles is still there, a skeleton, where one meeting a month is held...just enough activity to keep the building in "Church" status. Tax purposes, I Imagine. Not impressed.

Catholic Church didn't pan out, not being punny. As I left it from lack of fellow Catholic's rendered attection, I was chided that I was "playing with fire" and I was not to forget Catholic Dogma and the fact that there was a box of envelopes waiting for my pick-up...and that church fellowship was not only to be unexpected, but neither be pursued.

So we're Lutheran again.

Oh, and my Roman Catholic sponsor was quite right that our two-windowed basement apartment, one useful window, one not available to open, this one bedroom apartment, two doors from my childhood church (To where we all had returned exuberant), had a middle-of-the-night electrical fire: The cause; power bars and extension cords being used for inner-wall wiring. That Unforgettable Fire.

So now we're minimalists. Overnight. And born again to the faith that was once so all encompassing...now outwardly expressed to our fellow fellowshippers.

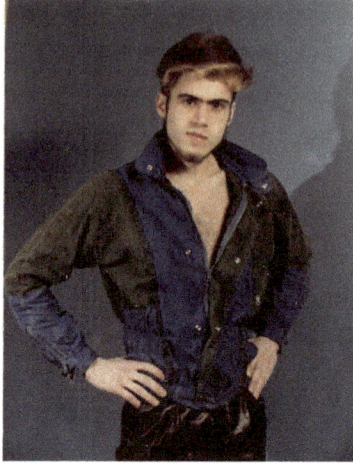

Chapter Five:
Staying alive.

So now, we are finally up to speed with everything past and traumatic. (Although there could be much more relivable gunk). Carlos Castaneda quoted his Mentor with a saying something like, "there is only life left to live." Brilliant. So is there anything past Schizophrenian? Yes and no. Medications are a control, a muting of impossible symptoms...they are not a cure. They used to say that if you had a full recovery, you probably were erroneously diagnosed to begin with. What a way to find out, trial and error, then thirty years of anguish. But I'm better for the first(?) time, seeing that I must have been better than psychotic at one point in my pre-schizophrenian career. Nobody worked harder or was more devoted to their vocation. And its elimination across the board.

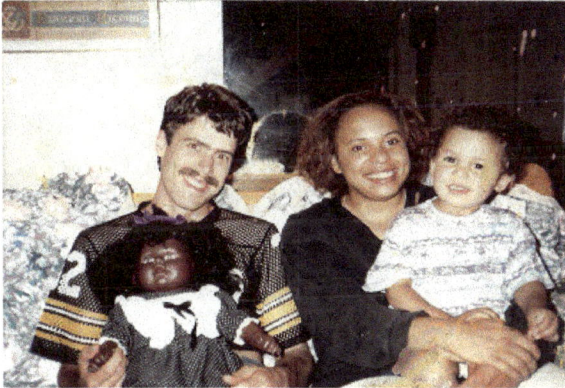

Some people go through three or four careers in a lifetime, provided that they don't careen. I've found the nature of this particular occupation, Schizophrenian, is akin to the dual qualities of light (both a wave and a particle)...so mental illness can show itself, but there is no precise pinpointing possible, since it can morph to a different quality at will. And there is nobody more intent to remain lame-brained than someone with an over developed inter cellular dialogue happening. We all know that we're special from the initial care given to us, onward. We only become more militant with the rejection of the general public, and maybe our family members' non-acceptance.

Things get worse. We are like aliens. Everybody knows that we exist, but few ever admit to seeing or encountering one in real life. We are the hysteria causers. Who would believe how human and sensitive we could be? To embrace us would mean to join our team, and scale that huge, sliver-thin chasm between them and us, solving myriads of difficulties immediately. So, like headless chickens, they scurry away, returning to their life

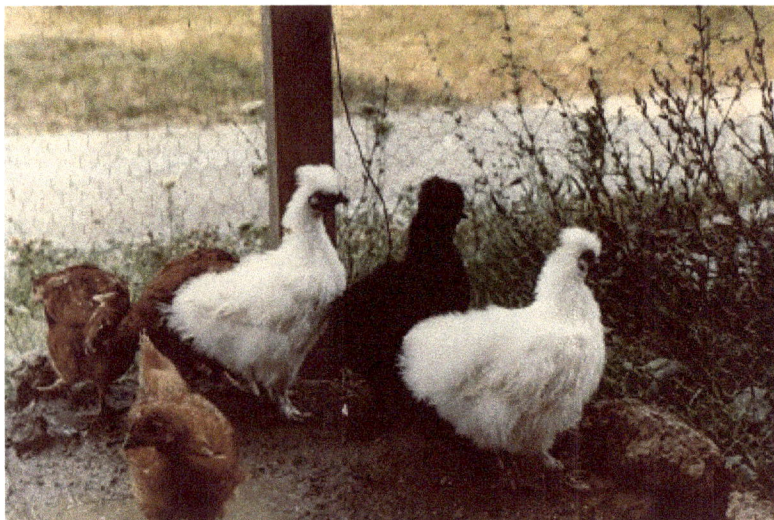

non-headless chickens

devoid of substantial thought-patterns. Truly, it is like you have to stop thinking in order to secure a place in University, a few degrees, an amazing job, a house, a spouse...and so there is no need for compassion returned, in this guise of a civil, social, all-embracing community.

I have had my moments, and for your information, aliens and schizophrenics DO exist.

When I was sixteen, I walked home from my job, a hefty five or eight miles, and when I got to a certain road, an urge came upon me to traverse down the middle yellow line. It took about ten or fourteen minutes. Not one single car, or truck, or bus, came onto this busy street until I was safely finished. In my magical way of thinking, that was my escape, my departure, my success.

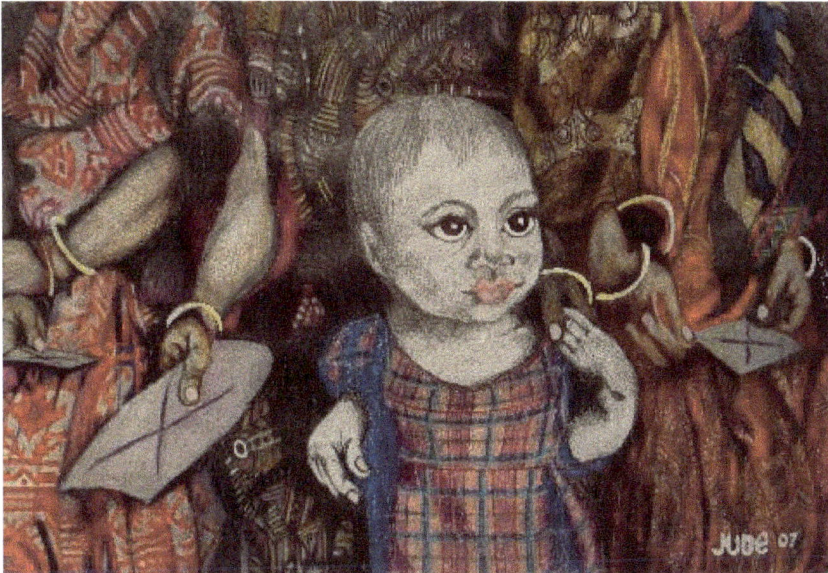

The original that sold, then was donated to the Salvation Army, and was bought back by me for ten bucks.

If you think I am crazy, you try it yourself. Wear one of those "X" shirts and runners that glow upon impact, in the middle of Inverness, a busy thoroughfare in Hamilton, on its yellow line. Oh, and it must be done at night, so bring those glow in the dark airplane directing sticks. Just keep mindful of the Police, obviously.

I must tell you that now, after explaining my stance towards life as "one of those ones", there is peace. I do not worry about whomever is angry with me by telepathy or the nearest floor-model color television, frowning away, to a catchy beat. The voices are long-gone with a few rare exceptions of intra-scullular anomalies. Occasional gibberish.

I am militantly deluded by my two grandkids, whom I maintain as being the cutest, most hilarious, well-behaved blonde babies that I have ever had the privilege to be the Gramma Banana of. And I feed them worms, of the gummy (candy) type. They shout out, in rhyme,

"If you're happy and you know it, clap…
Noooooo!!"

When I had shingles at age fifty two (why waste any time) I reported to Jimmy, my fave Grandson, that I had had a fight with a bear. He thought about it, considered that bears rarely get angry, especially at Gramma Banana, he thought some more. He looked at me compassionately and queried,"Why did the bear scratch you?" How do you answer that? An out-and-out lie badmouthing an innocent bear, that did not even exist. How do your synaptic gymnastics outsmart your own four year old grandson? By the way, do you even know what a grandparent is? Something so simple that even a small child can operate it. That's me. Claire Bear, my fave Granddaughter, has the odd, (in number, not patterned habit) sarcastic comment, amazingly advanced, especially comedic in her timing. I once, only once complemented Claire at her advanced math, counting to twenty-eight, "That's really good, Claire" Her smart-bottomed response I did not even hear, but it was something akin to, "Maybe for YOU"

My real Husband, George, still adores the parquet floors that I walk upon. I discovered whilst making my vows that this man that I was in the public process of marrying for life, had indeed been through much more pain than I.

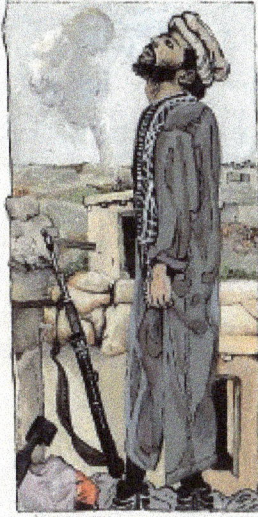

Afghan Man

And I didn't even notice, in all that time. So I faked it through my vows, wondering how I could have omitted such suffering in observing glances between puffs? What was my motivation after all? I think, as well as possible, that I was hoping to become famous in two years, then George would die, and I would be primed to meet Sting.

So, everybody, whenever I mention that man, I have discontinued my medications, or at least lowered my dosage. Unless you witness my well times when I am perfectly well-thinking to not really care one whit. I mean, pick up the phone, buddy.

And my Daughter has finally relinquished repaying me in installments, over my many, many mistakes, being "Mummy". Amanda is still the most beautiful creature on the planet, and her beauty has squelched any desire to remain sick, since she simply exists. What wonderful reasons to get better.

So, if you have made it this far in my testimony to living in reality, you will understand just what recovery is, broken glass and all. Thought-water all over the place. What IS a girl to do? Go on with her life, and keep grinning. Remember nobody, including the deluded, or psychotic, can SEE voices, even their own, anyway, so take a method-acting class, fake it until the weed starves out. And if you can, QUIT SMOKING anything weed-like! Cancerous tobacco, or its ugly, clever cousin, pot, or theater popcorn pulmonary wrecking vapes. If this is too hard to do, consider that moment of folly when you first lit up, because it was "cool". Good Luck. I haven't exactly quit, it being such a harsh word, I simply abstain. Indefinitely.

Chapter Six:

The Schizophoniks

In one of those dungeons called "Boarding Houses", Georgie and I met. He was highly musical and interested, I was artistic and musical and captivated. And George was not my first Rock Star but my favorite. We spent long hours getting to know each other through stolen glances. I guess that's what romance is. Sometimes. Our shyness and his remaining marriage marred any advances of the relationship romantically. So we sang. He initiated our career, in taking hold of the Children's Museum with typical dinosaur-loving five year old audiences. So not only did we sing, but I, myself contributed artistically in real-to-life dinosaur murals, indiscernible to the untrained post-toddler eye. They could have passed for the real thing.

The Schizophoniks name was initiated by our co-boarder named Joe whose family's praise worthiness consisted of transporting the church bell to The Basilica of Christ the King just before it was opened, and the naming of the main venue in Hamilton-Wentworth of the time, merely, "Hamilton Place". I guess that three's a charm because Joe coined the catchy title "The Schizophoniks" for our band, always downwards of three members.

Things moved fast. The Schizophoniks plowed ahead with disabled tirelessness. No thought could stand in our way. Okay, let's just say we did our best.

We started out humbly, seeing that I had a postpartum psychosis to wrestle with for a long while. Our gigs were frequent yet simple. We had no necessary time off for recording of successive albums. We did monthly birthday parties, one lasting for fourteen years of once a month singing. We sang for

Rainbow Ceramics and Gifts, at Halloween and Christmas, most of the audience being fellow Mentally "Inspired" ones, Rainbow being a sheltered workshop. One might initiate laughter at this point, but none of "Us" frankly care. A gig is a gig, And those performances were meant for therapy to the vulnerable members of this "Just Society" called Canada, remember? They, themselves loved our music...and we developed a rapport with the professionals, as well.

We belted out "Let it be" on a hot summer afternoon in a funeral parlor at a ceremony for one of us that did not quite make it. The place was hot, those in attendance were silent, and the doors and windows were wide. It was moving, but especially since this young man, a brother to all of us, had his own humble artistic gifts and gentle wisdom. Sadly gone.

But our priority was to leave this mess of a world a little better for Amanda, our young daughter, so, when we received a little bit of money from a family member's kindness, we immediately got the Grant Street Studio on the phone, booking one full day, at a painful one thousand dollars. We had five songs, four of them being original Larry Mersereau's, and the fifth, "No Woman, No Cry", a favorite of the entire planet, by Bob Marley. Our 'button-adjusting-guy' in that sound-proofed room was named Robin, and was an excellent production coach for us as well as an open ear for our testimony. We were just trying to raise money for Schizophrenia research, with one special child in mind.

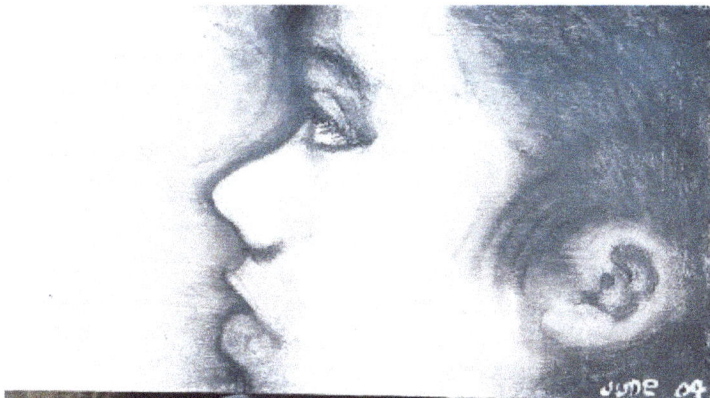

So, we began, and I honestly don't know how many cigarettes were smoked, or in what order we recorded song by song, but I do know that it took a good hour of gazing gold and other precious metallic albums until I identified one from, and I AM dropping names, the band known as U2, namely, the "Joshua Tree". And so, I said, perpetually intellectual, "I get it!"..."The Joshua Tree."

It proved to be a long exhausting day, so we stopped for a luncheon and education session for Robin, about the possible heights of success for even the most-humbly-beginning-ones-waxing-disabled. This culture has no words for "successful Schizophrenian." Most Schizophrenians who succeed, do it all in reverse. First fame, then money, then breakdown. We two, having broken down first are stuck singing in nursing homes, for the elderly. For free. For life.. But a gig is a gig.

Once the day finished, we had our tape to mass produce, which we did, one-by-one on our double tape-decked beat box. We made fifty copies by hand and sold all of them, the proceeds going to research. I think proceeds means whatever money was made after bills were paid, because somehow we broke even. My residual past-pregnancy fog could not compute. Where did the money go? Lessons learned, we kept our own personal brush with famous gold records quiet, quite glad that we did not brush too closely and knock the thing off the wall.

My Dad once met Bishop Tutu.

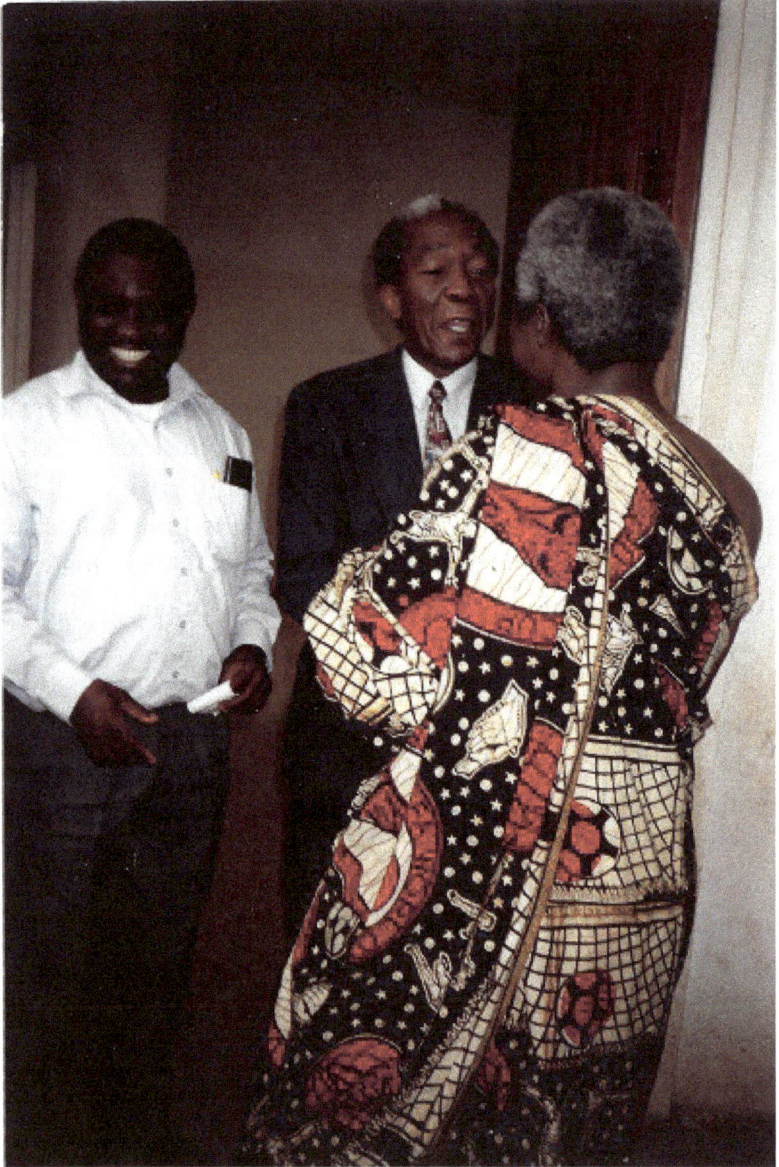

No caption required

And what follows the sighting of a famous record album in real life? The inauguration of T. Melville Bailey Park, naturally. Our career soared to singing "Country Roads", to a healthy 25 people present...some even appreciating country music. They immediately responded, we were getting good at music, and so, I introduced us as "The Schizophoniks" following with "We've been singing together for over three and a half...minutes" Banter and laughter. Good filler.

Anyway...we ended up recording in several studios, including the Cheese Factory, Aztec Studio, and a guy named John's basement studio for the formation of the "Emer" soundtrack. That occurred in Toronto, and we were treated to a lovely meal as payment at "Mr. Greenjeans" of the Eaton Center, downtown T.O. Yum.

Chapter Seven:

The Cottage Studio (Do you speak HUE?)

Color is a language. Do You speak Hue? was my coined phrase. And by now you have seen some of my original artwork for yourselves. Frankly, I prefer to write. And you know what? My wording is no longer cryptic nor condescending. (If you noticed, anyway). So where do we go from here...really?

George and I have done very well as pilgrims for Pilgrim Lutheran Church in our music and art. This Church is thriving with fellowship that defies any bad feelings ``left behind", since you can only have fellowship with your fellows. Now, knowing that there's no-one left to blame, Jeordy's challenge daily is to live constantly content at whatever comes our way. In a nutshell (pardon the pun)...I'm DONE!

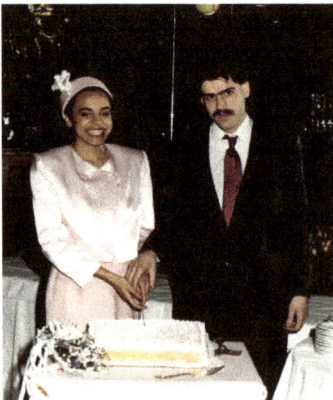

P.S."want some crushed nuts with that?

Paintings

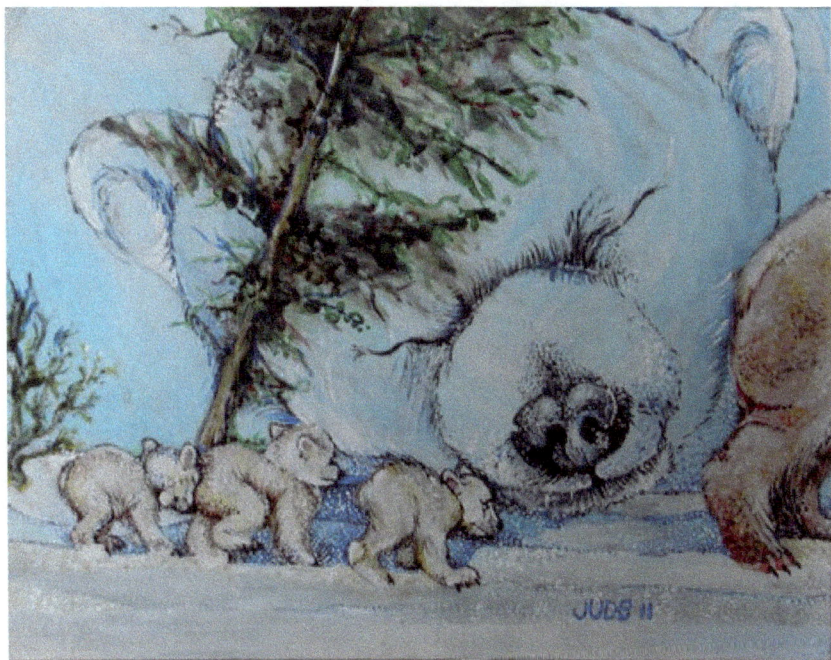

Grieving Grandmother

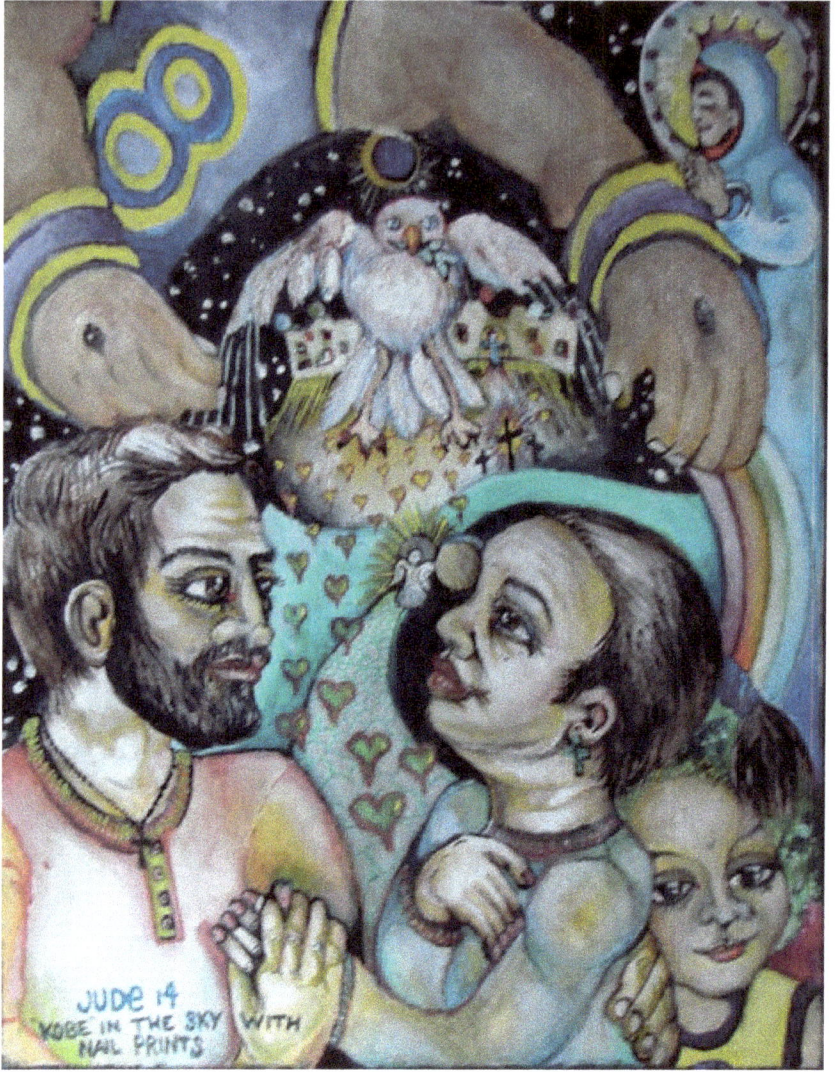

Kobe in the sky with nail prints

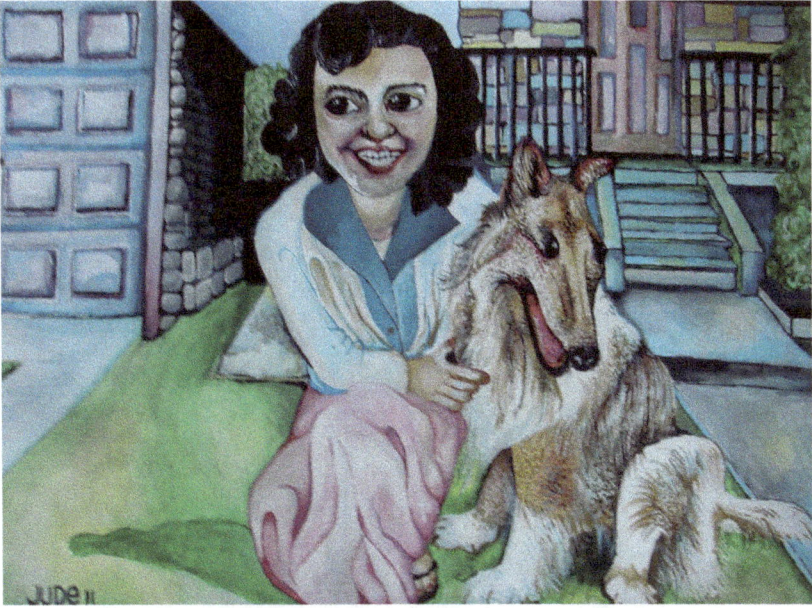

The Angelstone Princess

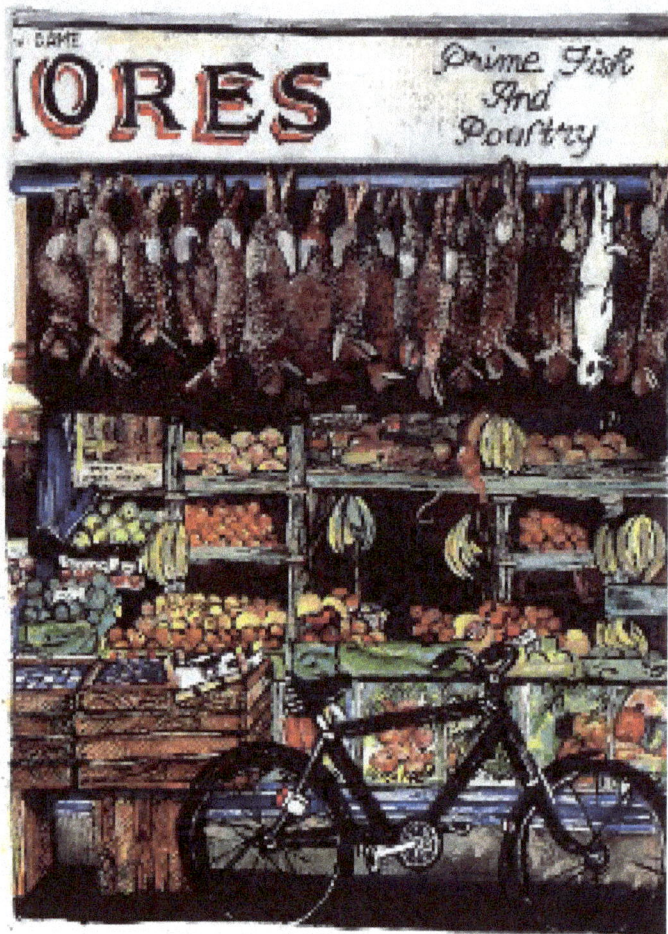

The English Market

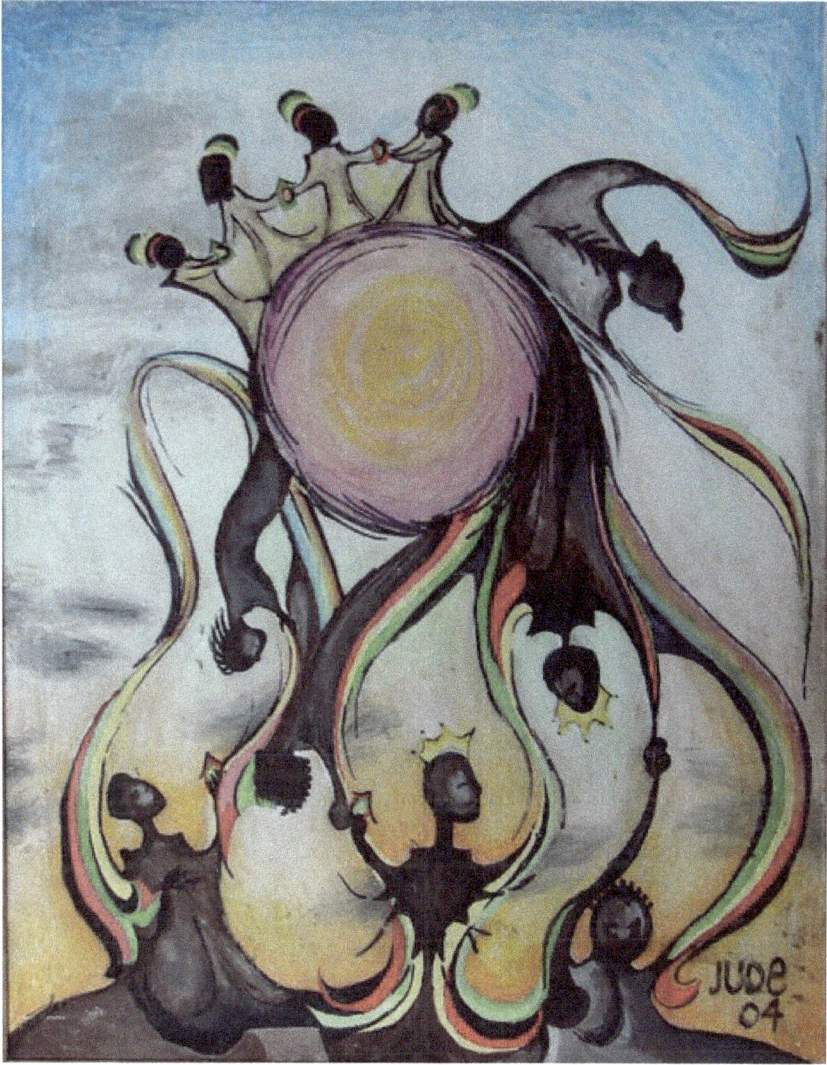

Sky Ribbons

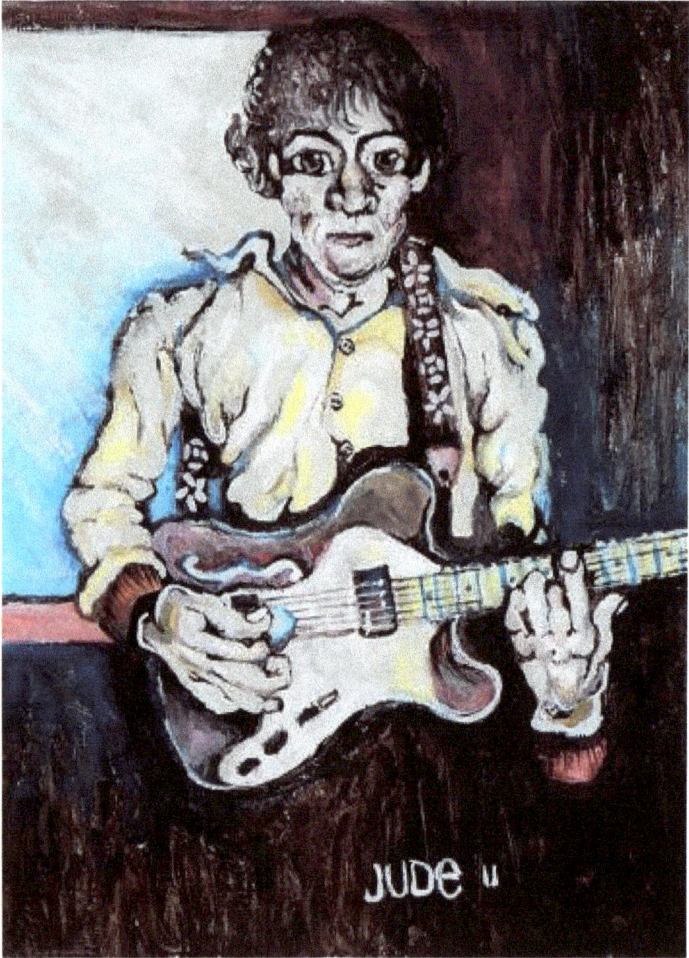

Georgie making the fire light

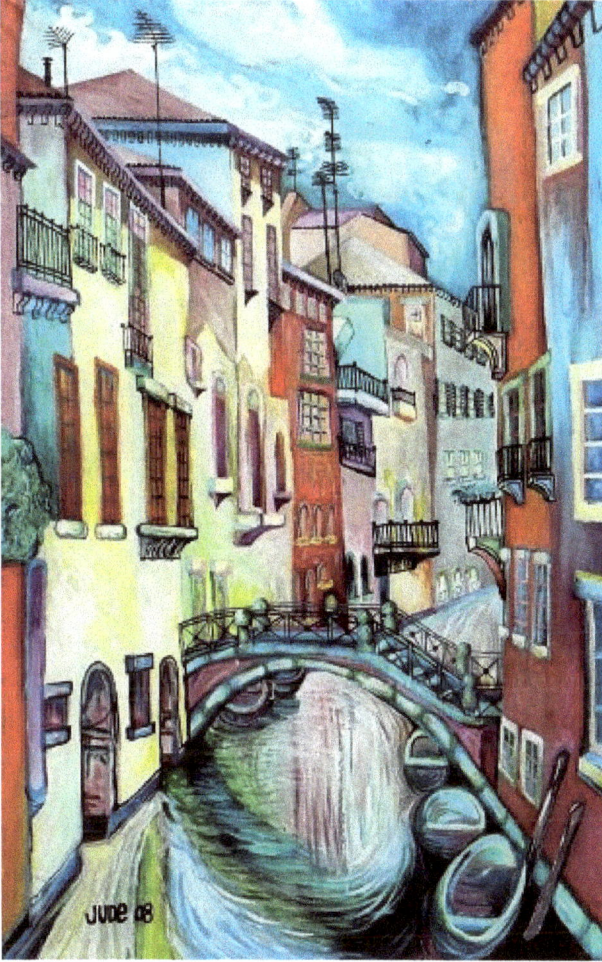

Very nice Venice

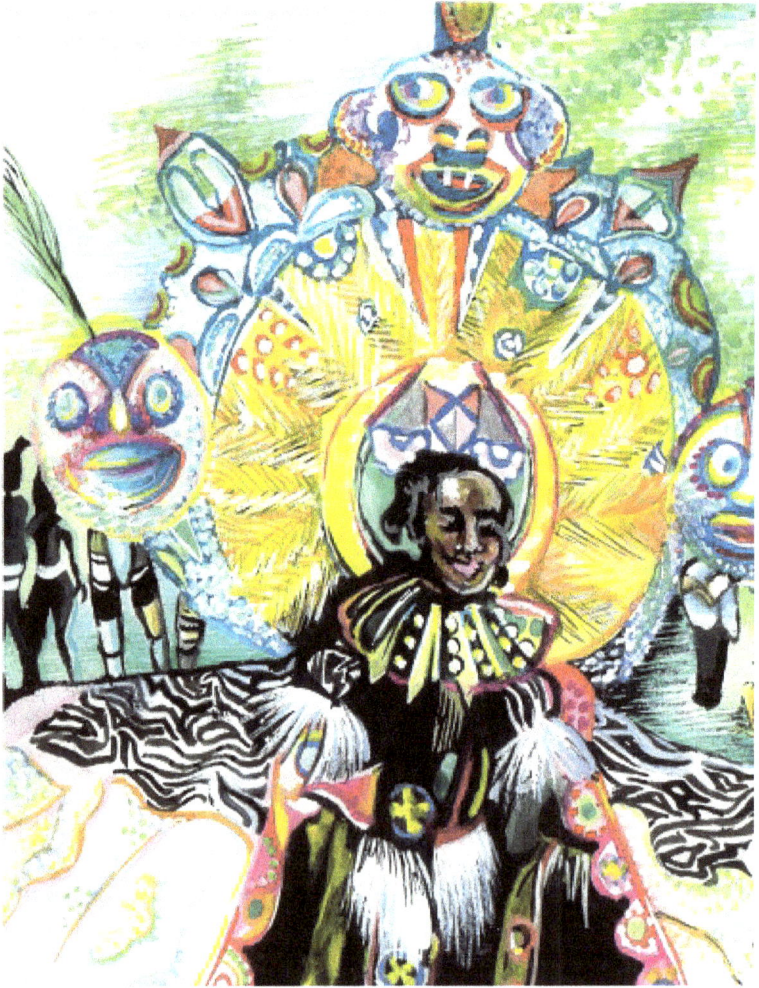

Caribana

ABOUT THE AUTHOR

Jude was born in Hamilton, Ontario, Canada on August 10, 1966 and graduated from Sir John A MacDonald High School in 1983 with an 87% average. Accepted at the College of Art in Toronto, she only attended briefly as she became ill in 1984/85. She married George on February 22nd/1989 and gave birth to their daughter, Amanda, January 14, 1990

Religion is very important to Jude who was baptized at the age of 4 and then confirmed on May 25, 1980. In 1999, she joined the United Church of Canada but in 2016, she converted to Catholicism. In 2018, she returned to the Lutheran Church and, as she says, became a born-again Lutheran.

Jude has always been involved in art and spent considerable time painting at the Cottage Studio in Hamilton – an art program for those with mental illness. She was one of three people profiled in a documentary done by Bridgeross called called, The Brush, The Pen and Recovery.

Jude also describes herself as hopefully happy although she can't recall how long she has been in that state.

Acknowledgments to the following:

...various helpful, empowering,emancipating hopeless sinners just like myself but without smacking of egocentricity

...thanks to Jack, for always outsmarting me, although in a completely unnoticed way; and May in her way of nurture

...appreciation to John, my art-adorer; and Monique, our best-bud par-excellence
...
...reciprocal steadfast approval to Barb and Guy,

...conversely, consistent converse stances from Mom and Dad Nunes' constructive discourse,

...thanks to the Lou people, the Lar people, the Stu people, for many, many patient rides home, quick quips, excruciating minutiae of affirming advice, and incessant laughter

...to Brenaomi, for being, Brenaomi,

...all the cousins and uncles and aunts, and nice nieces and nefarious nephews

...to Amanda, for always announcing, "MUMMY!"

...to Jimmy, our rock-star

...to Claire Marie amour, for always outsmarting me, although in a completely unnoticed way

...and everyone else, whomever you may be...for taking up space on this planet...just kidding...THANKS, y'all...I hope I've got that right.

jude

www.ingramcontent.com/pod-product-compliance
Lightning Source LLC
Chambersburg PA
CBHW070759100426
42742CB00012B/2190